Trusted advice

Your **healthy child**

A practical guide to over 80 childhood complaints

DRmiriam**stoppard**

LONDON, NEW YORK, MUNICH,
MELBOURNE, AND DELHI

Author's dedication: For Esmé, Maggie, and Evie

Revised Edition
Assistant Editor Dharini
Editor Bushra Ahmed
Senior Editors Saloni Talwar, Neha Gupta
Assistant Designers Niyati Gosain, Nidhi Mehra
Designer Anchal Kaushal
Senior Designer Tannishtha Chakraborty
Managing Editor Suchismita Banerjee
Design Manager Arunesh Talapatra
DTP Operator Vishal Bhatia
DTP Designers Pushpak Tyagi, Nand Kishor Acharya,
Mohammad Usman
DTP Manager Sunil Sharma
Picture Researcher Sakshi Saluja

Project Editor Daniel Mills
Senior Art Editors Isabel de Cordova, Edward Kinsey
Managing Editor Penny Warren
Managing Art Editor Glenda Fisher
Publisher Peggy Vance
Senior Production Editor Jennifer Murray
Creative Technical Support Sonia Charbonnier
Senior Production Controller Man Fai Lau

First published by Dorling Kindersley in 1998
Reprinted 2001, 2006, 2011

This revised edition published in Great Britain in 2011
by Dorling Kindersley Limited
80 Strand, London WC2R 0RL
A Penguin Company

Material in this publication was previously published
by Dorling Kindersley in *Baby and Child Healthcare* by
Dr Miriam Stoppard.

A CIP catalogue record for this book is available
from the British Library.
ISBN 978-1-4053-5650-3

Reproduced by Colourscan, Singapore
Printed in China by Leo Paper

Discover more at
www.dk.com

Contents

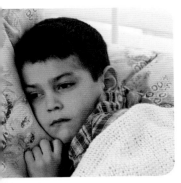

Introduction

It seems odd that there are so few books for parents that are devoted entirely to children's illnesses. Many baby books have a section on common childhood complaints, some even going so far as to include specific illnesses and their treatments; others approach the subject in a dictionary form, relying heavily on definitions but without giving very much background information and practical help to parents; indeed, very few treat the subject with the kind of detail, explanations, and guidelines that we have come to expect from similar books on adult diseases. Yet all parents worry about their children's health, and need the reassurance of a practical, easy-to-use guide; hence this book.

Here, more than 80 common childhood complaints are arranged in separate chapters by body system – for example, you will find bronchitis in the Respiratory system chapter, while nosebleed and stye are in the Eyes, ears, nose, throat, and mouth chapter – and form the mainstay of *Your Child's Health*. All the information is given in simple terms that are easy to understand. Parents are directed to possible courses of action in a clear, logical way, with step-by-step advice. Emphasis on speed is always made when it is important to contact a doctor or call an ambulance. An at-a-glance A–Z index of complaints is also included for emergency use.

Most childhood illnesses are minor, and others are easily preventable; inoculations are effective against most infectious diseases. In a baby, however, seemingly minor illnesses can cause complications: a cold that develops into a throat infection, for instance, may cause breathing difficulties. You will be understandably anxious if your child is sickening for something, is ill, or has had an accident. Sometimes deciding whether to seek medical help can be equally stressful. Even if your child's symptoms appear commonplace, you may worry that they are indicative of something more serious. You should never feel that you are being too cautious – if you find yourself wondering whether it is worth consulting the doctor, then you probably should. However, to help you determine the most likely causes of a complaint, most entries contain an at-a-glance symptoms box giving the most common symptoms of that ailment. In addition, each chapter begins with a simple diagnosis guide, which also gives the most common symptoms of the complaints covered in the chapter.

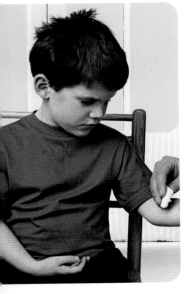

Your Child's Health has many useful illustrations; some will help with identification of symptoms, while others give practical tips in caring for a sick child. This is because one of my main aims is to give information in a readily accessible form, almost at a glance. There is, of course, ample opportunity to use the book as a straightforward reference guide so that you gain knowledge gradually. But more than this, an anxious parent faced with a sick child in the middle of the night needs straightforward, uncomplicated information and advice, and I have tried to arrange *Your Child's Health* in a way that I would like to see if I found myself in that position.

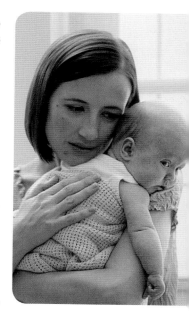

I don't have any personal axes to grind, but this book is opinionated and I make no apologies for this. However, where I have given an opinion, it is based on controlled research studies, or the lack of them, not on a purely personal basis.

Throughout the book the main aim remains the same: to give you enough clear, up-to-date information, backed up by your own instincts, to know when to be your own family nurse or doctor and when it is essential to get specialist medical help.

How to use this book

When your child is ill, you need to know what to do – whether to call the doctor or whether you can treat him at home yourself. You may also need help to determine the cause of the illness.

If your child is ill and you think you know the cause

Turn to the relevant illness entry later in the book (use the special A–Z listing on page 10 for speed and ease of finding if you're in a hurry). There you will find an explanation of the ailment in question, together with a list of the symptoms most likely to appear. The circumstances under which you should call the doctor are clearly defined, and are followed by a section detailing the most probable treatment the doctor will give. Most importantly, there is also advice on what you yourself can do to help your child.

If he has an obvious symptom of illness, but you are not sure which entry to look up, turn to the "Diagnosis guide" at the beginning of each chapter. (All the complaints are listed according to the system of the body that is affected – for example, bronchitis can be found in the "Respiratory system" chapter, while both nosebleed and stye are in the "Eyes, ears, nose, throat, and mouth" chapter.) Although it can be difficult to make a diagnosis on the basis of only one or two symptoms, these guides should help to point you in the right direction.

If you are looking after a sick child

The chapter "Caring for a sick child" on pages 11–22 gives tips on caring for your child when he is ill and shows, with photographs, how to

How to use the entries

Introduction
Gives a description of the complaint, explaining why it arises and how it is likely to develop.

Is it serious?
States whether or not the complaint is serious, and the conditions under which it would become serious.

How is it treated?
Tells you how to determine whether your child has a certain complaint or not, or it may suggest self-help measures that will provide relief while you contact the doctor. If the case is an emergency, this section will say so.

Should I seek medical help?
Explains the circumstances under which you should seek medical assistance.

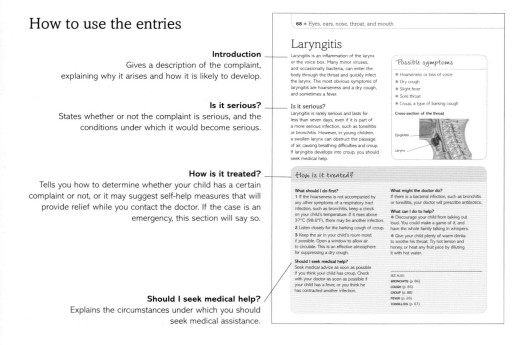

68 ✳ Eyes, ears, nose, throat, and mouth

Laryngitis

Laryngitis is an inflammation of the larynx or the voice box. Many minor viruses, and occasionally bacteria, can enter the body through the throat and quickly infect the larynx. The most obvious symptoms of laryngitis are hoarseness and a dry cough, and sometimes a fever.

Possible symptoms
- ✳ Hoarseness or loss of voice
- ✳ Dry cough
- ✳ Slight fever
- ✳ Sore throat
- ✳ Croup, a type of barking cough

Cross-section of the throat

Is it serious?
Laryngitis is rarely serious and lasts for less than seven days, even if it is part of a more serious infection, such as tonsillitis or bronchitis. However, in young children, a swollen larynx can obstruct the passage of air, causing breathing difficulties and croup. If laryngitis develops into croup, you should seek medical help.

Epiglottis
Larynx

How is it treated?

What should I do first?
1 If the hoarseness is not accompanied by any other symptoms of a respiratory tract infection, such as bronchitis, keep a check on your child's temperature. If it rises above 37°C (98.6°F), there may be another infection.
2 Listen closely for the barking cough of croup.
3 Keep the air in your child's room moist if possible. Open a window to allow air to circulate. This is an effective atmosphere for suppressing a dry cough.

Should I seek medical help?
Seek medical advice as soon as possible if you think your child has croup. Check with your doctor as soon as possible if your child has a fever, or you think he has contracted another infection.

What might the doctor do?
If there is a bacterial infection, such as bronchitis or tonsillitis, your doctor will prescribe antibiotics.

What can I do to help?
✳ Discourage your child from talking out loud. You could make a game of it, and have the whole family talking in whispers.
✳ Give your child plenty of warm drinks to soothe his throat. Try hot lemon and honey, or heat any fruit juice by diluting it with hot water.

SEE ALSO:
BRONCHITIS (p. 86)
COUGH (p. 85)
CROUP (p. 88)
FEVER (p. 26)
TONSILLITIS (p. 67)

take a temperature and give medicines. It also provides practical advice on how to reduce fevers and make your child comfortable, how to keep him amused, how and what to feed him, and, should the need arise, how to prepare him for a stay in hospital.

Using the entries

The illness entries are divided into a series of body-related chapters, and form the core of the book. They take two basic forms: in the majority of the entries, a detailed description of the illness is given, with a "Possible symptoms" box for easy checking, a list of what to look for first, and various treatments that might be given. In a few entries, where appropriate, the symptoms box is not given since the symptom itself is the complaint's name – for instance, dizziness, in the "Head and brain" chapter. Two special entries (fever and vomiting) form the basis

of so many common childhood illnesses that each one has a small symptoms chart of its own referring you to the various possible causes.

Within each entry, another section, "Should I seek medical help?", gives those instances where you should consult a doctor and also defines the urgency of the assistance needed. Emergency is just that, and you will be told to call an ambulance immediately or go straight to the nearest hospital emergency department; "Consult your doctor immediately" also indicates urgency and you should get in touch with him day or night to get his help; "Call your doctor as soon as possible" suggests some urgency but one that could await an early appointment during surgery hours; and lastly, "Consult your doctor for advice" indicates that the ailment is not serious, but that it is advisable to talk to your doctor about it.

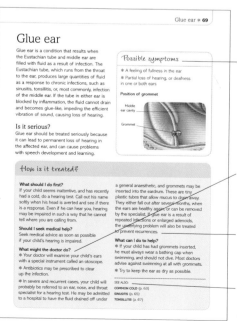

Possible symptoms
Lists the symptoms that are likely to occur with the given complaint. Your child may have some or all of them; he may or may not develop them in the order given, although that is the most likely sequence.

What might the doctor do?
Outlines the treatment most likely to be given to your child.

What can I do to help?
Makes suggestions as to what you can do to assist the doctor in the treatment of your child, and gives home treatment and nursing tips.

See also
A cross-referencing system to other entries. You may be referred to another complaint because it could be the possible cause of your child's complaint.

A-Z Guide to complaints

Although the complaints covered in this book are listed according to the part of the body affected, there are times when it becomes important to pinpoint something instantly. To get the most from the book, once you have identified the complaint, read the entry carefully, then follow the *What should I do first?* section. Your doctor will never mind being contacted if you are uncertain about symptoms. Always double-check instructions if any medication is prescribed.

Index of complaints

Chapter 1

Caring for a sick child

Caring for **a sick child** can be a nerve-wracking experience for any parent. The secret of coping is **understanding what to do and when,** and knowing when to call in the professionals.

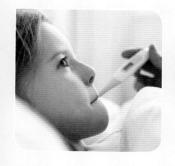
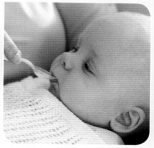
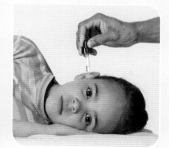

Calling for medical help

Most parents seem to know instinctively when their child is unwell or sickening for something: he may not be as lively as he usually is, he may refuse his food, he may become clingy, and so on. However, parents are not always able to diagnose exactly what is wrong, nor are they necessarily able to recognize whether the child's symptoms are serious or not, or even potentially serious. It's always worrying when a child is ill, and the situation can be even more difficult if you cannot decide whether or not to call for medical help. You know your child best, so if in doubt, call the doctor. There are some

circumstances, such as after a serious injury, when medical help should be sought immediately. For most parents, these situations are quite obvious. There are, however, many more situations where the seriousness isn't as clear-cut. This is where the worry comes in: "Are my child's symptoms normal or are they potentially serious?". What you must remember is that most doctors won't mind if you seek their advice.

Before calling make sure you have a note of what the doctor may need to know: a description of your child's symptoms, when they started, what order they occurred in, how severe they are, and whether anything precipitated them (has he eaten something poisonous, for instance). Your doctor will also want to know your child's age and medical history.

If your child is already having treatment from your doctor and you are worried about his progress, call your doctor again. If you need advice outside normal surgery hours, NHS Direct or your GP out-of-hours service will be able to help.

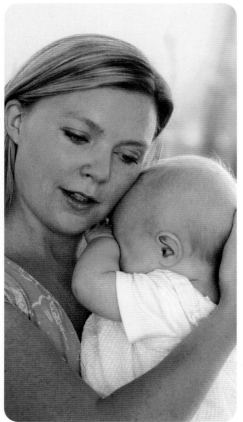

Your sick child Many children become more demanding when they are ill and want to be with their mothers all the time. While being as loving as possible, guard against starting habits you don't want to continue.

When to ask for medical help

Listed below are the circumstances under which you should seek medical help if you are concerned about your child. The following are all important signs, so never ignore them:

Temperature
* A persistently raised temperature of over 39°C (102.2°F) for more than six hours despite trying to bring it down.

* A raised temperature along with a seizure or if your child has had seizures in the past.

* A raised temperature accompanied by a stiff neck and headache.

* A temperature below 35°C (95°F) accompanied by a cold skin surface, drowsiness, listlessness, and lack of animation.

* A temperature that drops and then rises again suddenly.

* A temperature of more than 38°C (100.4°F), for more than three days.

Diarrhoea
* If your baby has diarrhoea for more than six hours.

* If diarrhoea is accompanied by pain in the abdomen, a temperature, or any other obvious signs of illness.

Vomiting
* If your baby has been vomiting for more than six hours.

* Dizziness with nausea and headaches.

* Nausea and vomiting accompanied by pain on the right side of the abdomen.

Loss of appetite
* If your baby goes off his food suddenly, or is less than six months old and doesn't seem to be thriving.

* If your child usually has a hearty appetite, but refuses all food for a day and seems listless.

Pain and discomfort
* If your child has headaches with dizziness.

* If your child complains of blurred vision, especially if he's recently had a bang on the head.

* If your child has severe griping pains, which occur at regular intervals.

* If your child has a pain on the right side of his abdomen and feels sick.

Breathing
* If his breathing is laboured and his ribs draw in sharply with each breath.

Emergency situations

Dial 999/112 for emergency help if you notice any of the following signs or symptoms:

* Your child has stopped breathing.

* Your child is breathing with difficulty and his lips are going blue.

* Your child is unconscious.

* Your child has a raised temperature and other signs of meningitis, such as drowsiness and a purplish rash.

* Your child has a deep wound that is bleeding badly.

* Your child has a serious burn (see p. 42).

* Your child has a suspected broken bone (see p. 110).

* Your child has a chemical in his eyes.

* Your child's ear drum or eye has been pierced.

* Your child has eaten a poisonous substance.

Temperature

In children, normal body temperature ranges between 36°C (96.8°F) and 37°C (98.6°F). Any temperature over 37°C (98.6°F) is classed as a fever. Hypothermia develops if the temperature falls below 35°C (95°F).

Body temperature will vary according to how active your child has been and the time of day: it is lowest in the morning because there is little muscle activity during sleep, and highest in the late afternoon after a day's activity. An abnormally hot forehead could be the first indication that your child has a temperature. To be accurate, however, you must take your child's temperature with a thermometer. Because the temperature control centre in the brain is primitive in young children, their temperature can shoot up more rapidly than in adults.

When your child has a fever, you should take her temperature again after 20 minutes, just in case it was only a transitory leap. Never regard a high temperature as the only accurate reflection of whether or not your child is ill; a child can be very ill without a high temperature or quite healthy with one.

Thermometers

There are two main types of thermometer: digital and ear sensor. Do not use a mercury thermometer with a child.

Digital thermometers are easy to use with children of all ages, and are safer to use than mercury thermometers because they are unbreakable. Digital thermometers are battery-operated, so be sure to keep spare batteries on hand.

Treating a raised temperature

The raised temperature that accompanies an illness is the body's way of responding to infection, and is a sign that the body is marshalling its defences (see p. 25). If your

Tips for taking temperature

✳ Never leave your child alone with a thermometer in her mouth.

✳ Never take your child's temperature if she has just stopped running about.

✳ Always read the manufacturer's instructions carefully.

✳ Digital thermometers are battery operated so be sure to keep some spare batteries on hand.

✳ Wash the thermometer after use in cool, soapy water.

✳ Always store the thermometer in its own case.

child has a high temperature, she will be very uncomfortable and irritable, so it is important that you lower her temperature. To do this, remove your child's clothes and blankets, and leave her covered by only a single cotton sheet. If her temperature rises over 39°C (102.2°F), she could be more comfortable left uncovered while wearing a short-sleeved cotton T-shirt and underpants, or a vest and nappy.

If your child's temperature is over 39°C (102.2°F) for longer than half an hour, and removing her bedclothes hasn't helped, try using a fan to cool the air temperature around her.

The most efficient way of reducing your child's fever is to give her medicine. Paracetamol and ibuprofen can both be given to children, as they have few side effects. They are available in liquid form, so are much easier to give to young children. Do not give either to your child for longer than two days without consulting your doctor.

Using thermometers

The armpit method is best for babies and very young children. Always wash a thermometer with cool, soapy water after it has been used. Store a thermometer in its own case and always keep it somewhere you can find it easily when you need.

Armpit method

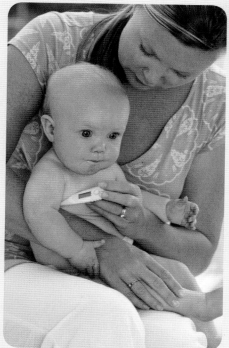

1 Hold the thermometer by the top end. Sit with your child on your lap, facing away from you. Holding the thermometer, raise your child's right arm so that you expose her bare armpit.

2 Put the thermometer into the armpit and lower her arm over it. Hold the arm down until you hear a "beep". Remove and read.

Note Temperature taken like this will be about 0.6°C lower than the actual body temperature.

Oral method

1 Ask your child to open her mouth and raise her tongue. Place the thermometer under the tongue.

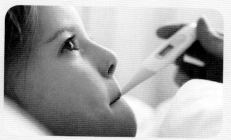

2 Ask your child to place the tip of her tongue firmly behind her lower front teeth – this will hold the thermometer in place. Then ask her to close her lips – but not her teeth – over the thermometer so that the seal is airtight. Check to make sure she is not gripping the thermometer with her teeth.

3 Leave the thermometer in your child's mouth until you hear a "beep". Remove and read the number in the window.

Using an ear sensor thermometer

Place the tip of the thermometer inside the ear for a reading. It reads in 1 second and you will hear a beeping noise. The sensor is easy to use and can be used while your child is asleep.

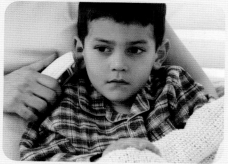

Medicines

When you take your child to the doctor, he may prescribe some form of medicine for him. Ask your doctor to give you as much information as possible about the medicine: ask if any side effects are likely, whether there are foods to be avoided or special precautions to be observed while your child is taking medication, and clarify if the medicine has to be given before or after a meal. Most medicines for children can be given with a spoon, syringe, or dropper. Droppers and plastic syringes are often more suitable for

babies who haven't learnt to swallow from a spoon. Some medicines for older children are supplied as tablets or capsules.

On most occasions your child will be co-operative, but there may be the odd time when he simply refuses to take his medicine. This is one instance when bribery is justified, so don't hesitate to give the medicine with a favourite food. Very occasionally, a child will resist physically. When this happens, there really is no alternative but for you to force them.

Giving medicines to a baby or young child

It can be more difficult to administer medicines to babies. You will need the help of another adult or an older sibling. Position your baby carefully so that he is slightly raised. Never lay him down flat while giving him medicine because he may inhale it into his lungs.

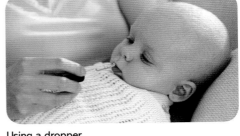

Using a dropper

1 Hold your baby as described left and take up the specified amount of medicine into the glass tube.

2 Place the dropper in the corner of your baby's mouth, and release the medicine gently.

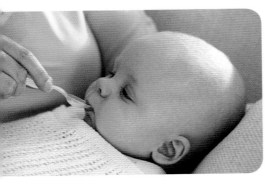

Using a spoon

1 If the baby is very young, sterilize the spoon by placing it in a sterilizing solution or by boiling it. Hold your baby in the crook of your arm. If he won't open his mouth, open it by gently pulling down his chin; if necessary get someone else to do this.

2 Place the spoon on his lower lip, raise the angle of the spoon, and let the medicine run into his mouth.

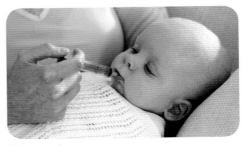

Using a syringe

Put the required dose into the syringe. Hold your baby as described left. Place the syringe in the corner of your baby's mouth, and release the medicine gently.

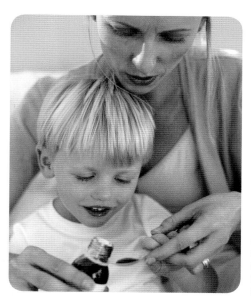

Giving medicines and tablets to older children

On the whole, children do not generally mind medicine too much, and often want to pour medicine out for themselves rather than let you give it to them. I have listed a few tips below that may help if your child is difficult. For example, tablets can be crushed and mixed with jam or ice cream. Capsules, however, should not be broken.

Helping your child take medicine
Older children will generally be happier taking medicine if they feel involved in the preparation, such as measuring out the doses.

Tips for giving medicines

Giving medicines to babies

* Enlist the help of another adult, or older brother or sister.

* If you are on your own, wrap a blanket around your baby's arms so that you can stop him struggling and hold him steady.

* Only put a little of the medicine in his mouth at a time.

* If your baby spits the medicine out, get the other person to hold his mouth open while you trickle the medicine into the back of his mouth. Then gently but firmly close his mouth.

Giving medicines to older children

* Suggest that your child holds his nose while taking the medicine, so lessening the effect of the taste.

* Don't hold your child's nose forcibly, as he may inhale some of the medicine.

* Mix liquid medicine with another syrup, such as honey.

* Don't add liquid medicine to a drink, as it will just sink to the bottom of the glass or stick to the sides and you won't be sure that your child has had the whole dose.

* Show your child that you have his favourite drink ready to wash the taste of the medicine away; do this even if you do not normally allow him to have this drink.

* Help your child to clean his teeth after taking any liquid medicine to prevent the syrup from sticking to his teeth.

* Crush tablets between two spoons and mix the powder with something sweet, such as honey, jam, or ice cream.

Medicines: continued

Giving drops

It is always easier to administer drops to a baby or young child for ear, nose, and eye infections if you lay him on a flat surface. If possible, get someone to help keep him still and hold his head steady. With an older child, ask him to tilt his head back or to the side while you put the drops in.

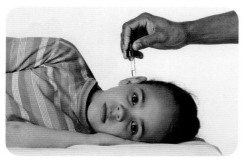

Ear drops

1 Lay your child on her side with the affected ear uppermost. (Hold a young baby in your arms.)

2 Put the drops into her ear, and hold your child steady until the drops have run into the canal.

Tips for giving drops

✳ Warm nose drops and ear drops by standing the container in a bowl of warm water for a few minutes, so that your child doesn't get too much of a shock when the liquid drops into his nose or ear.

✳ Be careful not to let the dropper touch your child's nose, ear, or eye, or you will transfer the germs back to the bottle. If the dropper does touch your child, make sure you wash it thoroughly before putting it back in the bottle.

✳ Proprietary drops should not be used for longer than three days without consulting a doctor – if they are used for too long, they can cause worse irritation and inflammation than the condition you were treating in the first place.

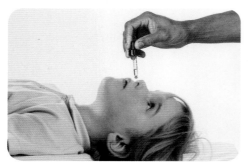

Nose drops

1 Tilt your child's head back and drop liquid into each nostril. (If you have a young baby, hold him in your arms).

2 Count the number of drops as you put them in. Two or three at a time are normally sufficient; any more will run down his throat and could cause him to cough and splutter.

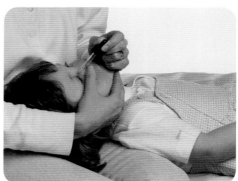

Eye drops

1 Tilt your child's head so that the infected eye is slightly lower, to prevent drops running into the healthy eye. Hold a young baby in your arms or hold an older child's head still with your free hand.

2 Very gently pull her lower eyelid down, and let the drops fall between her upper and lower eyelid.

Medicine cabinet

Always keep some medicines in the house in case of an emergency in the middle of the night when you may not be able to get to a chemist easily. Keep them somewhere obvious, so that you can find them quickly when you need them. Never mix different tablets up in the same container, and never keep any left-over prescription medicines. Keep all medicines well out of reach of children, in a high, locked cupboard, if necessary. You should also have a first-aid kit. Keep all the equipment in a clean, dry, airtight box, and put it somewhere it can be found quickly in an emergency.

The items listed in the box (see right) would all be useful to have in emergencies and are therefore well worth keeping in the house.

Medicines to avoid

The following items, commonly believed to be useful, should be avoided:

* Any proprietary product that contains aspirin. Aspirin must not be given to anyone under 16 years of age.

* Any proprietary product containing a local anaesthetic, such as amethocaine or lignocaine, because they can cause allergies. These are most generally found in creams for mouth ulcers or insect stings.
* Any skin creams containing antihistamines (unless prescribed by your doctor); they can cause skin allergies.
* Mouth washes, eye drops, nose drops, and ear drops, unless recommended by your doctor.

Useful household items

* Packet of frozen peas or ice cubes in plastic bags for cold compresses.
* Folded newspaper can make a splint to support a broken limb.
* Elastic belt to support a strained or sprained limb.
* Rehydration fluid to replace fluid lost during vomiting or diarrhoea.
* Vinegar to mix with water to soothe jellyfish sting.

Medicine cabinet

Your medicine cabinet should contain the following essential items, as well as a first-aid kit:

* Digital or ear sensor thermometer
* Paracetamol tablets or liquid paracetamol
* Liquid ibuprofen
* Calamine lotion

First-aid kit
* Box of adhesive dressings
* Wound dressings – cotton wool and gauze pad already attached to a bandage

* Mild antiseptic wipes
* Cotton wool
* Gauze dressings – keep dry and paraffin-coated ones
* Surgical tape
* Crepe bandages for supporting sprains and strains
* Triangular bandage
* Safety pins, scissors, and blunt-edged tweezers

Nursing a sick child

Few parents escape being called upon to look after a sick child – all children fall ill at some time. Babies often become very clingy, and may cry more than normal because they do not understand what is happening to them. If a baby is being breastfed he will probably want to be fed more often, for the comfort of being near you. Bottle-fed babies will also want to be cuddled, and will want smaller feeds more often. If your baby has recently given up his bottle, you may find that he wants it back again.

Older children can also become rather insecure when they are ill, and often want to be with a parent all the time. Nursing a child requires love and patience. Simply use your common sense. If you are worried, see a doctor (see pp. 12–13). If any medicines are prescribed, make sure you give them exactly as directed, and follow any nursing tips your doctor gives you.

Tips for nursing your child

* Use cotton sheets – they are much more comfortable for a child with a temperature.

* Change his sheets regularly, particularly if he has a fever – clean sheets feel better.

* Let him get up if he does not want to stay in bed all the time, but put a jumper on over his pyjamas and make sure he's wearing socks or slippers.

* Leave a box of tissues for his use on his bedside table.

* Leave a bowl beside your child's bed if he is feeling sick so that he doesn't have to run to the toilet. If he vomits, hold his head and comfort him, and give him a strongly flavoured sweet, or help him clean his teeth, to take away the after-taste.

Should my child stay in bed?

Take your lead from your child about whether or not to keep him in bed. There's no real need to keep a child with a fever in bed, although he should stay in a draught-free room where the temperature is kept constant. The room does not have to be particularly hot – if it is comfortable for you, it should be warm enough for him. If your child is really ill, he will probably want to stay still, and will sleep a lot, but when he is awake he will want to be with you, so make up a bed for him in the room where you are working so that he can hear and see you. If he wants to be out of bed and playing, let him do so in the corner of the room. Leave his bed straightened so that he can lie down when he wants to. If he is very tired, it is better to put him to bed, but remember to visit him regularly so that he does not feel neglected.

Should I isolate my child?

Most evidence suggests that, in cases of infectious diseases, the degree of severity of the disease increases if there has been sustained close contact. It is therefore advisable to keep other children away from your infected child as much as possible. Obviously, if your child has a more serious infection that needs isolation, such as meningitis (see p. 118), your doctor will arrange for him to be admitted to hospital or advise you on the necessary precautions. If your child has rubella (see p. 31), you should warn any women you think may be pregnant or who may come in contact with someone who is pregnant.

Feeding a sick child

Most children with a fever don't want to eat, so although you should offer food, you should never force your child to eat if he seems unwilling. As long as he is getting plenty of liquids, he can survive perfectly well for two or three days on very little. When the illness is over, your child's appetite will return.

Getting a sick child to drink

While your child can survive without much food when he is ill, it is important that he drinks as much as possible to replace any fluid lost in sweating, vomiting, or diarrhoea. A fevered child needs to drink at least 100–150ml (3–5fl oz) liquid per kilogram (2lb) of body weight per day, or 200ml (7fl oz) per kilogram (2lb) if he is vomiting or has diarrhoea. Get him to drink as often as you can; help an older child by leaving his favourite drink by the bed. Fizzy glucose drinks are neither nutritious nor necessary; I do not recommend them.

Occupying a sick child

When your child is ill you can legitimately spoil him. Let him play with games that were previously forbidden in bed. Even messy activities such as painting will not cause too much mess if you put a large sheet of polythene over the bed.

Be easy on yourself as well, and relax all the rules on tidiness – you can always clear up later. Sit down and spend time with him: read him stories, play games, or help him with his colouring. Let him watch television while he is ill – have the television in his room or in the room where you are both sitting. Buy him some new toys. If he isn't too ill, wrap them and play a game with the parcel; ask him to guess what's in it and let him tear off the wrapping. Ask his friends to come and see him and let them play for a short time. If your child is not in bed all the time, there's absolutely no reason to keep him indoors on a warm day, even if he has a mild fever, but don't let him exercise too strenuously. If he wants to stay outside for longer than a few minutes, he is probably getting better anyway.

Feeding and drinking tips

Feeding your child

* Give your child small meals more often than you would normally.

* Don't scold him for not eating – he will eat again as soon as he gets better.

* Give your child his favourite foods.

* If your child has a sore throat, give him ice-cream or an ice lolly made with fruit juice or yogurt to soothe it.

* If your child is feeling slightly sick, give him mashed potato.

Making drinks more interesting

* A sure ploy is to offer drinks in a tiny glass or an egg cup. It is more fun and makes the quantities look smaller.

* Give your child fresh fruit juices and dilute them with fizzy mineral water to make them more exciting.

* Use an interesting straw such as a curly or bendy one.

* If your child does not like milk, make it more attractive by adding milkshake mixes or ice-cream. Try varying the drinks sometimes.

* With a young child or baby, get him to sip drinks from a teaspoon. You could make it into a game by using a long-handled spoon.

Getting better

As your child gets better, his appetite will start to come back and he will be more active. As soon as his temperature is back to normal in the morning and evening, he is probably ready to go back to school, although, if he has been suffering from an infectious illness, it may be wise to check with your doctor first. A young child may have regressed slightly while he was ill. For example, if he was just out of nappies, you may have to start potty training again. Try not to worry about this too much.

Your child in hospital

You will be doing your child a great favour if you encourage her to think about hospitals as friendly places. Try taking her with you if you are visiting a family friend or relative – provided the person does not mind and visiting regulations allow it.

Preparing your child

If your child has to go into hospital, for an operation for example, and you are given some warning, prepare her by discussing as many aspects of her stay as possible. Talk about it with the rest of the family as well and get her generally used to the idea.

Answer all her questions honestly. She will probably ask you if there will be any pain or discomfort after the operation. If you say that nothing is going to hurt and it does, she will simply get a shock and will not trust you in the future. Explain that there will be some discomfort but that it won't last long.

Another good way to prepare her for a hospital stay is to read her a book about someone who goes into hospital. You could also buy her a toy stethoscope and play doctors and nurses with her. Encourage her to be the doctor or nurse and suggest that she make up a hospital bed for her favourite teddy bear or toy.

In hospital

Few children's wards are frightening places. However, hospitals have found that it is very important for parents to be with their children as much as possible while they are in hospital and, because of this, almost all of them now allow parents to stay with their child, particularly if the child is very young. Many hospitals have sleeping facilities for parents with children. When you are there, ask the ward sister and nurses how you can help with the daily routine.

What to take into hospital

If you can, you and your child should pack her case together a few days before she has to go in.

* ✳ Three pairs of pyjamas
* ✳ Dressing gown and slippers
* ✳ Three pairs of ankle socks
* ✳ Hairbrush and comb
* ✳ Sponge bag with soap, flannel, toothbrush, and toothpaste
* ✳ Bedside clock
* ✳ Portable music player with headphones
* ✳ Favourite books and portable games
* ✳ Favourite picture or photograph to put by her bedside

You will be encouraged to bathe and change your child, help with her feeding, and play games with her. If the ward has a teacher, ask if you can help with your child's schoolwork. If she is well enough, ask her own teacher to give you the work she would normally be doing at school.

If you cannot be with your child all day, try to make some arrangement so that someone she knows well is with her all the time.

Back home from hospital

It's quite normal for a child to behave a little oddly when she comes out of hospital. First, your child's sleeping and eating patterns may have changed – she may tend to do both earlier than usual. Secondly, because your child has been away from her domestic discipline, she may make a fuss about small points such as brushing her teeth. Don't be too hard on her at first, give her time to readjust to being at home before you insist that she fits in with the old routine.

Chapter 2

Infectious diseases

Infectious childhood illnesses are less common now than they once were, thanks to immunization, but they still occur. This chapter gives you advice to enable you to help your child through them.

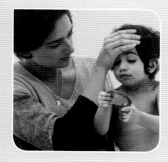
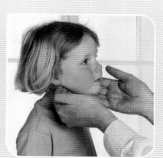
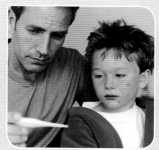

Diagnosis guide

Children will always catch infectious diseases, so it is important to be able to identify and treat them when they occur. To use this section, look for the symptom most similar to the one that your child is suffering from, and then turn to the relevant entry. See also p. 13 for a list of symptoms requiring emergency treatment.

Blotchy red rash starting behind the ears and spreading elsewhere, with swollen neck glands, possibly **Rubella** (see p. 31)

Red-brown rash starting behind the ears and spreading elsewhere, usually preceded by a runny nose and sore eyes, possibly **Measles** (see p. 28)

Aches and pains with swollen glands and a rash behind the ears, possibly **Glandular fever** (see p. 30)

Intensely itchy small blisters in clusters appearing first on the trunk, then the rest of the body, possibly **Chickenpox** (see p. 27)

Headache with fever and a rash, possibly **Measles** (see p. 28) or **Chickenpox** (see p. 27)

Swelling on either or both sides of the face, possibly **Mumps** (see p. 29)

Swollen neck glands with sore throat accompanied by a fever, possibly **Glandular fever** (see p. 30) or **Tonsillitis** (see p. 67)

Symptoms of infectious diseases

SYMPTOMS	COMMON CAUSES
Your child has a cough and a runny nose.	She possibly has a **Common cold** (see p. 63).
Your child has a cough, sore throat, and aches and pains.	She may have **Influenza** (see p. 87).
Your child has a sore throat and difficulty in swallowing.	She may have **Tonsillitis** (see p. 67), **Laryngitis** (p. 68) if her voice is hoarse, or **Glandular fever** (see p. 30) if her neck glands are swollen.
Your child has a rash of itchy, red spots starting on the trunk.	She may have **Chickenpox** (see p. 27).
Your child had a runny nose and sore eyes, and now has a brownish-red rash.	She possibly has **Measles** (see p. 28).
The sides of your child's face and the area under her chin are swollen.	She possibly has **Mumps** (see p. 29).
Your child's ears are painful, or if she is too young to tell you, she cries and tugs at her ear.	She possibly has a middle ear infection or **Earache** (see p. 70).
Your child has diarrhoea.	She could have **Gastroenteritis** (see p. 98), or **Food poisoning** (see p. 99).
Your baby or child is breathing rapidly and with great difficulty.	**Seek medical help immediately.** She may have **Bronchitis** (see p. 86) or **Croup** (see p. 88).
Your child cannot bend her neck without experiencing pain, and turns away from bright light.	**Seek medical help immediately.** Your child may have **Meningitis** (see p. 118).

Fever

The range of normal body temperature is 36–37°C (96.8°F–98.6°F). Anything over 37°C (98.6°F) is a fever, although the height a temperature reaches is not necessarily an accurate reflection of the seriousness of the sickness. Seek medical help if your child's temperature is high for more than six hours, despite trying to bring it down. A fever is not in itself an illness, but rather a symptom of one (see p. 25). Apart from any illness, your child's temperature will reflect the time of day and activity level: after a very strenuous game of football, for example, her temperature could temporarily be over 38°C (100.4°F).

Is it serious?

A fever is always serious in a baby under six months old. If the temperature remains high, there is a risk of the child having a seizure.

How is it treated?

What should I do first?

1 If you suspect that your child has a fever, take her temperature (see p. 15), then check it again 20 minutes later.

2 Put your child in bed, remove most of her clothing, and cover her only with a light sheet, even if the room is cool.

3 Use a fan to cool the air around your child.

4 Give the recommended dose of paracetamol. Never give aspirin to a child under the age of 16.

5 If needed, ibuprofen can be given instead of paracetamol.

6 Encourage your child to drink small amounts of fluid at regular intervals to prevent dehydration.

Should I seek medical help?

Get medical advice promptly if your child is under six months old. Also seek help immediately if your child has a seizure, has had one in the past, or if seizures run in the family; if the fever lasts for more than six hours despite trying to bring it down; or if you are worried about any of the other symptoms.

What might the doctor do?

If the cause of fever is a bacterial infection, your doctor or nurse will probably prescribe antibiotics. If it is an ailment such as chickenpox or a common cold, no medication will be given, just advice on how to make your child comfortable.

What can I do to help?

✷ Place a cold compress or a wet face cloth on your child's forehead.

✷ Don't wake your child to take her temperature. Sleep is important.

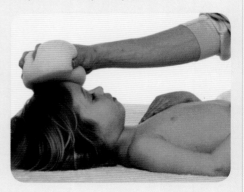

SEE ALSO:

CHICKENPOX (p. 27)
COMMON COLD (p. 63)
MEASLES (p. 28)

Chickenpox

Chickenpox is a very common infectious childhood disease. It has an incubation period of between 17 and 21 days, and causes only mild symptoms. Some sufferers may have a headache and a fever, although the majority give no real indication of illness at all except for the characteristic itchy chickenpox spots.

These spots cover most parts of the body and can even appear in the mouth, anus, vagina, or ears. They develop every day for three to four days, and quickly create blisters that leave a scab. Your child is infectious until the scabs have dropped off. The spots may leave shallow scars when they heal.

Is it serious?

Chickenpox is not a serious illness. However, in rare cases, the chickenpox virus may cause encephalitis or be complicated by a condition known as Reye's syndrome.

Possible symptoms

* Small blisters developing every day for three to four days, usually starting on the trunk, then spreading to the face, arms, and legs, and eventually scabbing over
* Intense itchiness
* Headache and fever

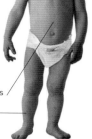

Sites of rash

Early sites

Later sites

How is it treated?

What should I do first?
1 Damp down the itchiness by applying calamine lotion to the rash, or by giving your child warm baths in which you have dissolved a handful of bicarbonate of soda.

2 As far as possible, keep your child away from other children; don't send her to school until the scabs have all dropped off.

Should I seek medical help?
Seek medical advice as soon as possible to confirm that your child has chickenpox. Check with your doctor if the spots become red and swollen, which indicates infection; or if your child can't stop scratching; or if she is feverish or complains of neck ache when the spots have scabbed over and she should be feeling better.

What might the doctor do?
* Your doctor or nurse will prescribe an antibiotic if any of the spots is infected.
* An antihistamine cream may also be prescribed.

What can I do to help?
* If your child is still in nappies, change them frequently and leave them off whenever possible to allow the spots to scab over.
* Cut your child's fingernails short and discourage her from scratching.

SEE ALSO:
BLISTERS (p. 41)
ITCHING (p. 35)

Measles

Measles is an infectious childhood disease, caused by a virus, which is now rare since routine immunization was introduced. It is very contagious, and has an incubation period of between eight and 14 days. The first indications of measles are usually symptoms similar to those of a common cold, with a fever that keeps rising, and small, white spots that form inside the mouth on the lining of the cheeks (Koplik's spots). Your child's eyes may also be red and sore. The initial symptoms are followed three days later by small, brownish-red spots behind the ears; these spots merge together to form a rash over the face and torso.

Is it serious?

Measles is a deeply unpleasant childhood illness, but it is normally not serious. However, in rare cases your child may develop complications, such as infection of the middle ear or pneumonia.

Possible symptoms

* Runny nose and dry cough
* Headache
* Fever, as high as 40°C (104°F)
* Small, white spots inside the mouth
* Red, sore eyes, intolerant of bright light
* Brownish-red rash of small spots, starting behind the ears and spreading to the torso

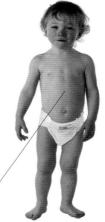

Rash starts behind the ears, and spreads to the torso

Sites of rash

How is it treated?

What should I do first?

1 If your child has a fever, try to bring it down with paracetamol or ibuprofen.

2 If your child's eyes are sore, bathe them with cool water.

3 Make sure he drinks plenty of fluids by offering him small amounts regularly.

Should I seek medical help?

Consult your doctor immediately if your child gets worse after seemingly recovering, or if he complains of an earache.

What might the doctor do?

* Your doctor or nurse will advise you to keep your child in bed for as long as his temperature remains high. He will examine your child's ears to check that there is no ear infection. If there is, he may prescribe a course of antibiotics.

* Your doctor may prescribe eye drops for your child's eyes if they are sore.

What can I do to help?

* Don't send your child back to school until the rash has faded.

* Check that any other children are immunized against measles.

SEE ALSO:

COMMON COLD (p. 63), **EARACHE** (p. 70), **FEVER** (p. 26)

Mumps

Mumps is an infectious childhood disease, which is now rare since routine immunization was introduced. It mostly affects children over the age of two. It is caused by a virus, and has an incubation period of 14 to 21 days. Your child will seem generally unwell for a day or two before the major symptoms appear. The salivary glands in front of and beneath the ears and chin swell up, and there may be a fever. The swelling can appear first on one side of the face, then the other, or on both sides at once, and may cause pain when swallowing. He will complain of a dry mouth because the salivary glands stop producing saliva.

Is it serious?

Mumps is a mild disease. However, if before, during, or after swelling, your child has a severe headache and stiff neck, this could be encephalitis or meningitis, which are serious.

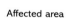

Possible symptoms

* Swollen, painful testes in boys, lower abdominal pain in girls

* Swelling of the glands on either or both sides of the face, just below the ears and beneath the chin

* Pain when swallowing

* Dry mouth

* Headache

* Fever

Affected area

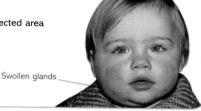

Swollen glands

How is it treated?

What should I do first?

1 Check your child's temperature to see if he has a fever. If he has, try to bring it down with paracetamol or ibuprofen.

2 Liquidize his food if he is having difficulty eating, and give him plenty to drink. Encourage him to rinse out his mouth to alleviate the dryness.

3 Put your child in bed with a hot-water bottle wrapped in a towel to hold against the affected side.

Should I seek medical help?

Get help to confirm the diagnosis, if your son's testes are painful or your daughter has abdominal pain. Check immediately if, after 10 days, your child's condition has worsened and he has a headache and stiff neck.

What might the doctor do?

* There is no specific treatment for mumps. Keep your child off school until five days after the swelling has gone down.

* If the testes or ovaries are swollen, your doctor or nurse will advise bed-rest until the swelling has subsided, and will probably prescribe paracetamol to relieve pain.

What can I do to help?

Be inventive with liquid foods, such as egg-enriched milk shakes, soups, and yogurt.

SEE ALSO:
FEVER (p. 26), **MENINGITIS** (p. 118)

Glandular fever

Glandular fever, or infectious mononucleosis, is a viral infection that starts in much the same way as influenza, possibly with a rash similar to that of rubella. It is fairly common, affecting mostly teenagers and young adults; children can also contract it, but they tend to be less severely affected. There is no known cure for glandular fever, and it has to run its course – usually, about a month. In reaction to the infection, the glands become swollen, and the spleen may become enlarged. This does not in itself give rise to unpleasant symptoms, and the spleen returns to normal once the infection has gone.

Is it serious?

Glandular fever is not usually serious, but as so many of its symptoms are similar to those of other illnesses, you should seek medical help.

Possible symptoms

✳ Swollen glands, most commonly in the neck, accompanied by a fever

✳ Depression and lethargy

✳ Rash that starts behind the ears, spreading to the forehead

✳ Aches and pains

✳ Runny nose

✳ Sore throat

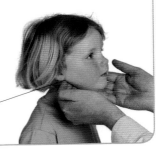

Checking for glandular fever

Check for swollen glands

How is it treated?

What should I do first?
1 Many early symptoms are similar to those of other ailments, but be alerted if the neck glands are swollen and there is a fever. Check your child's temperature regularly if her glands are swollen. If it remains high, give her paracetamol or ibuprofen.

2 Keep her isolated until you have a confirmed diagnosis, as the virus is infectious.

Should I seek medical help?
Consult your doctor immediately if you suspect your child is not just suffering from influenza or a common cold.

What might the doctor do?
Your doctor or nurse will take a blood sample. Glandular fever can be diagnosed with certainty only by finding antibodies in the blood. If the

diagnosis is positive, you will be advised to keep your child indoors and let her have plenty of rest; no further treatment is required.

What can I do to help?
✳ Don't send your child back to school until the doctor allows it.

✳ Keep your child indoors until the fever subsides.

✳ If she has a temperature, offer her plenty of fluids to prevent dehydration.

✳ The virus may reappear in the two years after the first attack, so look out for any symptoms.

SEE ALSO:

COMMON COLD (p. 63), **FEVER** (p. 26), **INFLUENZA** (p. 87), **RUBELLA** (p. 31), **SORE THROAT** (p. 66)

Rubella

Rubella, or German measles, is a mild infectious disease that is caused by a virus. It is now rare since routine immunization was introduced. It is contagious, and has an incubation period of 14 to 21 days. The rash usually starts behind the ears before spreading to the forehead and the rest of the body. It looks more like a large patch of redness than a series of spots. The rash lasts about two to three days and is rarely accompanied by serious symptoms, just a mild fever and enlarged glands at the back of the neck. The main danger with rubella is not to your infected child, but to any pregnant woman who may contract the disease from your child. Rubella can cause birth defects, such as blindness and deafness.

Is it serious?

Rubella is not serious, but keep your child in isolation for five days after the rash appears. It carries a slight risk of encephalitis.

Possible symptoms

* Slightly raised temperature
* A rash of tiny pink or red spots, which usually starts behind the ears before spreading to the forehead and then to the rest of the body
* Enlarged, swollen glands at the back of the neck and behind the ears

Site of swollen glands

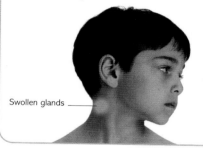

Swollen glands

How is it treated?

What should I do first?

1 Make sure that any woman who might be pregnant and has been in contact with your child is promptly informed of the infection.

2 Keep your child away from public places where he is likely to come into contact with pregnant women and other children.

3 If your child's temperature rises above 38°C (100.4°F), give him paracetamol or ibuprofen.

4 If your child is feeling unwell, put him in bed.

Should I seek medical help?

Check with your doctor to confirm that your child has rubella. Consult your doctor or nurse immediately if your child complains of a stiff neck or a headache.

What might the doctor do?

There is no treatment for rubella, but you will be advised to alert any women you know who might be pregnant, particularly those in the first four months of their pregnancy, if you haven't already done so.

What can I do to help?

Make sure that all the children in your family are immunized against the disease.

SEE ALSO:

FEVER (p. 26)

MENINGITIS (p. 118)

HIV/AIDS

HIV is a viral infection caused by the human immunodeficiency virus (HIV) that destroys the white blood cells in the body's immune system. The infection can lead to AIDS (Acquired Immune Deficiency Syndrome), which is a long-term debilitating illness. There are now drug treatments available to combat HIV and counter AIDS. Most HIV-infected children contract the virus from their mothers.

However, not all HIV-positive mothers will transmit the virus to their fetus, and there are also some ways of reducing the risk before and around the time of the baby's delivery.

HIV infection produces few symptoms initially, but as it develops into AIDS, the immune system weakens allowing diseases such as pneumonia to develop. Some infected children will show symptoms before they are two years old, although some may not show any signs until they pass the age of five. Anti-retroviral drugs have now improved the outcome of the disease to a great extent.

Possible symptoms

* Failure to thrive
* Recurrent diarrhoea
* Enlarged lymph nodes
* Frequent infections
* Attacks of pneumonia
* Developmental delay

Should I get medical help?

If you believe that your child is at risk of infection with the HIV virus, seek your doctor's advice immediately. Children who are HIV-positive need a high level of medical care.

What can be done?
* With your consent, a blood test will be performed to determine whether your baby is HIV-positive. Newborn babies of HIV-positive mothers can be difficult to diagnose, because they do not show any symptoms of the virus, but their mother's antibodies may be present in their blood for at least a year.

* If your child has the virus, anti-retroviral drugs will be prescribed to attack it, and to slow the development and progress of the disease.

* If you are HIV-positive, you will be advised not to breastfeed your child, as there is a small but important risk that you might transmit the virus to your baby via your milk.

* You will be referred to specialist organizations that can provide counselling and advice on how to manage the illness.

FOR HELP, ADVICE, AND DETAILS OF CENTRES
IN YOUR AREA, CONTACT:
The Terrence Higgins Trust
314–320 Gray's Inn Road
London WC1X 8DP
THT Direct 0845 12 21 200
Website www.tht.org.uk
Email: info@tht.org.uk

Chapter 3

Skin, hair, and nails

Minor ailments such as **bruises and stings** are usually easily taken care of; but **burns and bites** can be serious. This chapter takes you through the possibilities and provides **practical help** to see you through.

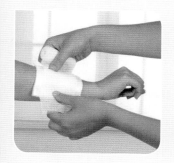
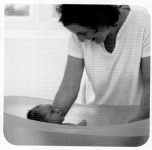
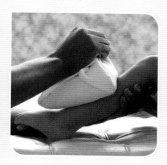

Diagnosis guide

Young children will get minor skin, hair, scalp, and nail problems, but fortunately most are easily treated and cured. To use this section, look for the symptom most similar to the one that your child is suffering from, or complaining of, then turn to the relevant entry. See also p. 13 for a list of symptoms requiring emergency treatment.

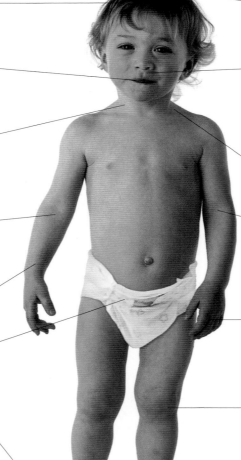

Yellow scales on your baby's scalp, possibly **Cradle cap** (see p. 50)

Small cracks on the lips, possibly **Chapping** (see p. 45)

Faint red rash over the neck, face, shoulders, and in the skin creases, with a flushed appearance, possibly **Heat rash** (see p. 44)

Itchy red or grey patch that extends out in a ring, possibly **Ringworm** (see p. 56)

White, itchy lumps in crops, possibly **Hives** (see p. 53)

Pimply red rash on the nappy area, possibly **Nappy rash** (see p. 49) or **Thrush** (see p. 121)

White blistered, itchy skin between the toes, possibly **Athlete's foot** (see p. 54)

Pain and redness on the toenail, possibly **Ingrowing toenails** (see p. 59)

Itchy head with small eggs clinging to the hair, possibly **Lice** (see p. 57)

Tiny, itchy blisters around the lips, possibly **Cold sores** (see p. 48), or that ooze and crust over bright yellow, possibly **Impetigo** (see p. 55)

Painful red lump filled with pus, possibly **Boils** (see p. 47)

Small puncture mark, possibly bee or wasp **Insect stings** (see p. 40)

Fine, short, itchy lines in the skin usually between the fingers, possibly **Scabies** (see p. 58)

Dry, scaly skin with a red rash mainly on the face, hands, wrists, ankles, and knees, possibly **Eczema** (see p. 51)

Numb, swollen blue skin that is itchy, possibly **Chilblains** (see p. 46)

Flat white or brown lump on the sole of the foot, possibly **Verruca** (see p. 60)

Itching

Itching is nearly always a symptom of some underlying skin problem, such as eczema or ringworm, the result of an infestation (scabies, fleas, or worms), sensitivity to some foodstuff or drug, skin contact with an irritant (hives), or the result of an infectious disease, such as chickenpox. Sometimes tension and worry can also cause itching, and scratching can make the itchiness even worse.

Is it serious?

Itching is rarely serious, but it should not be ignored.

How is it treated?

What should I do first?

1 To determine the cause of itching, the site may give you a clue. For example, itching around the anus and genitals could indicate worms or thrush; itchiness in the hair, lice; on the feet, athlete's foot; or between the fingers, scabies.

2 Check any pets your child comes into contact with for fleas.

3 Check to see if your child has eaten any new foods recently.

4 Note whether your child is taking any new medicines.

5 Try soothing the itching with calamine lotion, or give your child a cool bath.

Should I seek medical help?

Get advice as soon as possible if you can find no apparent reason for the itching, or if your child is having difficulty sleeping properly because of constant itchiness.

What might the doctor do?

* Your doctor or nurse will examine your child to determine the cause of itching. If the itching is a symptom of a particular condition, your child will be treated accordingly. Antihistamine tablets, liquid paracetamol, or an antiseptic cream may be prescribed to ease the itching.

What can I do to help?

* Dress your child in cotton underwear, so that fabrics such as wool and nylon, which irritate, do not touch his skin.

* If you have recently changed your washing powder or fabric conditioner, change back to the old brand and see if the irritation subsides. Rinse clothes well.

* Use a mild soap and shampoo for your child.

* To stop your child from scratching, put mittens on his hands whenever possible, and keep his nails short, to prevent infection should he break the skin by scratching too hard.

SEE ALSO:

ATHLETE'S FOOT (p. 54)

CHICKENPOX (p. 27)

CHILBLAINS (p. 46)

ECZEMA (p. 51)

HIVES (p. 53)

RINGWORM (p. 56)

SCABIES (p. 58)

THRUSH (p. 121)

Cuts and grazes

Small cuts and grazes can be treated at home, and should be cleaned up and possibly dressed to prevent germs from causing infection. Dress with a piece of sterile gauze held in place with adhesive tape, so that the air can get to the wound; plasters can also be used to dress a cut.

If the cut is a deep one, a few stitches might be necessary, and if there is a lot of blood loss, shock might follow.

Are they serious?

Small cuts and grazes are not serious. However, there is a risk of infection.

How are they treated?

If the wound is bleeding

1 Press the wound firmly to compress the ends of the damaged blood vessels, and raise the injured area above your child's heart.

2 Help him lie down. Keep the injured area raised, and press on the wound for up to 10 minutes.

3 Cover the wound with a sterile dressing or a non-fluffy dressing larger than the wound itself, still keeping the injured area raised above the heart. Secure the dressing with a firmly tied bandage. If blood seeps through, secure another dressing with a bandage on top. If necessary, support the wounded area in a sling.

If the wound is a small cut or graze

1 Sit your child down and gently wash the cut or graze with soap and water, making sure you remove all dirt or grit. If this causes a little fresh bleeding, press the wound with a clean pad.

2 Dress the wound with a plaster that has a pad large enough to cover the injury. Do not cover with cotton wool: fluffy materials stick to a wound and delay healing.

Should I seek medical help?

Take your child to the nearest emergency department if the wound is large and the bleeding persists after 10 minutes of pressure, the wound is very deep, the wound is on the face or is gaping, if there is dirt or a foreign

object in the wound that you can't get out, if the wound is deep but has only a small puncture hole in the skin, or if your child was playing in an area where animals are kept and the wound has been contaminated by dirt or grit. Check with your doctor if, after a day or two, you notice any red streaks extending from the centre of the wound as this could be a sign of infection.

What might the doctor do?

✳ Your doctor or nurse will clean the wound and stitch it, if necessary; any wound on the face will be stitched to minimize scarring.

✳ If the bleeding doesn't stop, a blood vessel may have been lacerated, and this will be tied off under an anaesthetic.

✳ If there is a deep wound, or a wound contaminated with dirt, your child will be assessed for tetanus, and may need a booster immunization.

✳ If there is an infection, antibiotics may be prescribed.

What can I do to help?

Change the dressing as instructed.

Bites

Most children love the company of animals, but because they are not always as gentle with them as they should be, bites can and do occur. The most common animal bites – from household pets, such as dogs and cats – leave puncture marks; humans leave teeth marks. Insect bites leave a weal resembling hives – a white centre on a red base. They are extremely itchy, but the pain and localized reaction usually fade within three to four hours. The bites of the common flea, normally from a household pet, also leave itchy weals.

Are they serious?
Animal, human, and insect bites, if untreated, can become infected.

How are they treated?

What should I do first?
1 Reassure your child and calm him down. If he has been bitten by a dog or a horse, for example, it is important that he does not remain afraid of these animals throughout his childhood. Try to persuade him that it is an isolated incident.

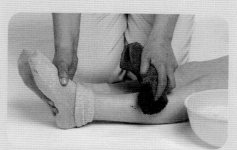

2 For animal and human bites, wash the wound with soap and water to remove any blood, saliva, or dirt. Put a clean dressing over the wound.

3 For insect bites, apply calamine lotion to relieve the irritation.

Should I seek medical help?
Get medical advice as soon as possible to check that an animal or human bite is not infected, and doesn't carry the risk of rabies or tetanus. Take your child to the nearest emergency department if the wound is bleeding heavily. Check with your doctor if, after 12 hours, the area looks red and swollen.

What might the doctor do?
* Your child may need to be immunized against tetanus.

* If your child's wound is infected, your doctor or nurse may prescribe antibiotics.

What can I do to help?
* You must emphasize to your child the need to treat animals carefully and not to tease them. In most cases, if a pet causes the injury, it will be an isolated incident and you should not try to get rid of the animal. If you are travelling abroad, be prepared for any problems by carrying a first-aid pack, and updating tetanus boosters before you go.

* You will need to clean the carpet, curtains, and furniture if you suspect that your child has been bitten by fleas. Flea powder to dust furnishings is available from vets and pet shops. Treat your pet, too.

* If your child is being bitten by mosquitoes, apply an insect repellent to his skin or clothes, or spray the room with an insect repellent.

SEE ALSO:
HIVES (p. 53)

Bruises

A bruise is a purplish-red stain in the skin, usually resulting from a blow or a knock that ruptures the small blood vessels near the skin's surface. It usually takes 10–14 days for a bruise to disappear completely; as it fades, it changes colour to maroon, then green or yellow as the blood pigments break down and are reabsorbed by the body. Resting, cooling, and holding up the affected part will soothe any pain.

Are they serious?

A bruise is rarely serious. If a bruise appears without any reason, this could relate to rare but serious conditions such as leukaemia and haemophilia.

Possible symptoms

✳ Purplish-red mark on the skin, which fades to maroon and then green or yellow

✳ Tenderness for a day or two

✳ Swelling if the bruise is over a bone

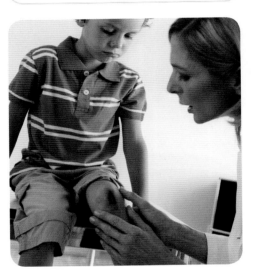

Minor bruises Comfort and reassurance are the best remedies for minor bumps and bruises.

How are they treated?

What should I do first?

1 A minor bruise needs no treatment at all, just a cuddle and reassurance if your child is upset.

2 If the bruise is large, apply a cold compress for half an hour or so. This will contain the bruising to some extent.

Should I seek medical help?

Take your child to the nearest emergency department if pain on the site of the bruise gets worse after 24 hours; an underlying bone could be broken. Check with your doctor if a bruise appears spontaneously with no apparent cause.

What might the doctor do?

✳ Very rarely recurrent bruising or bruises that appear spontaneously could indicate haemophilia or leukaemia. Your child may need to be referred to a specialist clinic.

SEE ALSO:
BROKEN BONES (p. 110)

Splinters

A splinter is a tiny sliver of material that becomes embedded in or under the skin. It may be wood, metal, glass, or a thorn.

Are they serious?

A splinter is very rarely serious, although it can often be painful and uncomfortable. Most splinters can be removed quite easily at home, but occasionally they are deeply embedded or difficult to dislodge. In such cases, seek medical help.

Occasionally splinters can cause deep wounds. Such wounds can be serious, particularly if they do not bleed much, because they carry the risk of infection, as splinters themselves are rarely clean.

How are they treated?

What should I do first?

1 Find out from your child, if possible, what material is embedded in the skin. If it is glass, the entire surface of the splinter will be capable of cutting into your child's flesh, so don't try to remove it yourself; seek medical aid.

2 If the splinter is not glass and the end is sticking out of the skin, remove it with tweezers. Sterilize them by passing the ends through a flame, then allow to cool.

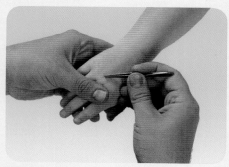

3 Grip the splinter with the tweezers as close to the skin as possible. Pull it out at the same angle it went in.

4 Squeeze the wound to make it bleed and flush out any dirt. Clean the area with soap and water. Dry it well, and cover with a dressing.

5 If you experience any difficulty while trying to remove a splinter, abandon the attempt and seek medical help.

Should I get medical help?

If the splinter is under the skin, do not try to remove it yourself. Seek medical help if the splinter is glass, or if it's contaminated with garden material (which increases the risk of tetanus). You should also seek medical advice if you cannot remove the splinter easily yourself.

What might the doctor do?

✳ If the splinter is deep in the skin, your doctor or nurse will remove it under a local anaesthetic.

✳ If there is any garden material in the wound, your child may need a tetanus booster injection.

Insect stings

Most stings cause only local irritation and pain. Bee and wasp stings make a small puncture hole in the skin; bees leave their stings behind, but wasps rarely do.

Are they serious?

A sting is rarely serious. However, if it causes an allergic reaction with severe swelling leading to loss of consciousness, if the sting is in the mouth or throat, or if your child is stung by a number of insects, then it should be treated as an emergency.

Possible symptoms

✳ Small puncture mark, with or without the sting left behind

✳ Localized swelling and irritation

✳ Breathing difficulties

✳ Signs of shock – rapid pulse, clammy and pale skin, shortness of breath, sweating, and faintness

How are they treated?

What should I do first?
Keep your child as calm and still as possible to slow the spreading of the poison.

If your child is stung by a bee or a wasp
1 If the sting is still in the skin, scrape it off. Avoid squeezing the sac because this will force more poison into your child's body.

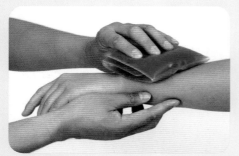

2 To reduce the pain and swelling, lay on a cold compress. Don't rub the area.

If the sting is in the mouth or throat
1 Give her cold water to drink, or an ice cube to suck. Call 999/112 for emergency help.

2 If the area swells quickly, lay her down on her side.

Should I seek medical help?
Take your child to the nearest emergency department if she has an allergic reaction, has been stung more than once, you can't remove the sting, or the area is swelling. Dial 999/112 for emergency help if she develops shock or breathing difficulties, or if she has been stung in the throat or mouth.

What might the doctor do?
✳ If your child has suffered an allergic reaction, your doctor or nurse may prescribe antihistamine tablets or cream, depending on the severity. Your child may also be given a series of desensitizing injections to prevent the same reaction in future.

✳ Your doctor or nurse will give drugs to control any swelling if your child has been stung in the mouth or throat.

What can I do to help?
✳ Make up an emergency pack of antihistamine medication if your child suffers an allergic reaction to insect stings. Carry it with you on holidays and outings.

Blisters

A blister is a fluid-filled bubble of skin that forms as a result of burns or friction, or as a result of exposure to extremes of temperature. Blisters vary in size, depending on the cause, and their purpose is to form a cushion to protect the new layer of skin growing underneath. The fluid is eventually reabsorbed by the body, and the outer surface dries out and peels away, leaving the healed skin behind. If the blister is broken before healing has taken place, there is a risk of infection.

Are they serious?
A blister is not usually serious.

Cleaning blisters When cleaning a blister, be careful not to burst it as this increases the risk of infection.

Possible symptoms

* Raised surface of the skin, filled with fluid, which may be as large as several centimetres across

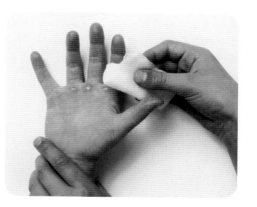

How are they treated?

What should I do first?

1 Don't prick a blister that has formed as a result of friction, burning, or extremes of temperature; leave it intact.

2 Protect blisters where friction may cause them to burst. For example, if the blister is a result of ill-fitting shoes or wearing shoes without socks, change your child's shoes for the time being, put two pairs of socks on your child, or use special blister plasters to protect the blister.

3 If the blister bursts, keep it clean and dry, and cover it with a gauze dressing or a blister plaster with a pad large enough to cover the whole blister.

Should I seek medical help?

Consult your doctor as soon as possible if the blister is large, or the result of a scald or sunburn. Consult your doctor as soon as possible if the area becomes infected, that is: if the blister becomes pus-filled; if red streaks extend outwards from it; if the skin surrounding it becomes red, tender, or swollen; or if your child complains of pain.

What might the doctor do?

* If the blister is infected, antibiotics may be prescribed.

SEE ALSO:
BURNS (p. 42)
COLD SORES (p. 48)
SUNBURN (p. 43)

Burns

A burn is an injury to the skin following exposure to heat, such as fire or electric current. The severity will depend on the situation and the cause. In a superficial burn, there may be just a reddened patch on the skin or a blister; in a deep burn, layers of skin may actually be removed.

Are they serious?

Apart from very superficial ones, all burns should be treated seriously, but electrical burns should be treated with particular caution because they may appear minor but can be deep. All burns should be assessed by a doctor because no matter how minor a burn may seem to be, there will always be some damage to the underlying tissue. (In deep burns, especially, there may not always be pain, because nerve endings may have been damaged by the burn.) All burns ooze a colourless liquid (serum), and if too much is lost your child could go into shock.

Possible symptoms

* Raw, red areas
* Fluid-filled blisters
* Small, blackened patch on the skin after an electric shock

How are they treated?

For small, superficial burns

1 Cool the affected area by placing it under cold running water for 10–15 minutes, or until the pain has gone.

2 Cover with a sterile dressing extended beyond the injured area. Don't apply creams or lotions, and certainly not butter or fat. Give your child liquid paracetamol or ibuprofen to relieve the pain.

3 Raise the affected part slightly, so that blood flow to the area is slowed down. This will help ease the pain.

For deep or electrical burns

1 If the burns were caused by a liquid, use a cloth to prevent it from getting on to your skin, and take off any of your child's clothing that the liquid has soaked into. Don't remove any clothing sticking to the skin.

2 If your child has suffered an electric shock, first break her contact with the electricity by turning off the current or moving her away with a non-conducting material, such as wood.

3 Cool the affected area by running cold water over it for as long as possible. If it covers a large area, put your child into a cool bath.

4 Cover the affected area with a sterile dressing. Don't apply any creams, lotions, butter, or fat.

5 To prevent shock, lay your child down with her legs raised and supported. Wrap her in a clean sheet to reduce the risk of infection.

Should I seek medical help?
All burns should be assessed by a doctor.

What might the doctor do?
If the burn is infected, your doctor will prescribe an antibiotic.

SEE ALSO:
BLISTERS (p. 41)

Sunburn

Sunburn is inflammation of the skin caused by excessive exposure to the harmful ultraviolet rays in sunlight. It always happens due to misjudgement or carelessness on the part of the parent. The best cure for this is prevention. Even adults should give their skins a chance to gradually acclimatize to the sun. It is necessary to be strict with children who may not appreciate the dangers. Your child's sunburn can result in tender and damaged skin that may blister or even peel off. Even in mild sunshine, the effects of the sun can be increased if you are near water, snow, or sand, where the rays are reflected off the bright surface.

Possible symptoms

- ✳ Red, hot, tender skin
- ✳ Blisters
- ✳ Itchiness prior to peeling skin

Is it serious?

If a large area of your child's skin gets sunburned, it can be very serious. The skin may lose its ability to regulate body temperature effectively, and as a result heatstroke may occur. Sunburn also poses a major long-term risk of skin cancer.

How is it treated?

What should I do first?

1 Apply a soothing lotion, such as calamine, to any tight and red skin to cool it down and reduce the irritation.

2 When your child is inside, don't put any clothing on the sunburned areas; leave them exposed to the air. Cover the sunburned areas properly when she is outside.

3 If blisters appear on the sunburnt patch, and your child complains of pain, give her paracetamol or ibuprofen. Take her temperature to see if she has a fever. If it is over 39°C (102.2°F), get medical help, and try to reduce the fever by fanning your child.

4 Keep your child out of direct sunlight for at least 48 hours.

Should I seek medical help?

Get medical advice if blisters form on your child's sunburned skin and she is feverish. Dial 999/112 for emergency help if your child has a fever but her skin is dry, and she seems confused and drowsy; it could be heatstroke, which should be treated as an emergency.

What might the doctor do?

✳ In a mild case of sunburn, your child may be given a soothing cream.

✳ If your child is suffering from heatstroke, she will be treated accordingly.

What can I do to help?

✳ Draw the sheets on your child's bed tightly, so that nothing scratches her tender skin.

✳ To prevent sunburn, keep all but the toughest parts of your child's skin covered up for the first few days of bright sunlight. Whenever she is in the sun, apply a total sunblock lotion to all the exposed parts of her body, and protect the nape of her neck with a wide-brimmed hat.

✳ Remember to apply sunblock lotion again after your child has been swimming.

✳ Keep a check on your child's skin, and if it is starting to burn, cover her up immediately.

Heat rash

Heat rash is a faint red rash in the areas of the body where the sweat glands are most numerous – on the face, neck, and shoulders, and in the skin creases, such as the elbows, groin, and behind the knees. It is quite common in babies because their sweat glands are still primitive and not efficient at regulating body temperature. Heat rash is not due to exposure to sunlight, but arises when the body becomes overheated and the skin responds with excessive production of sweat.

Is it serious?

Heat rash is never serious.

Possible symptoms

Areas affected

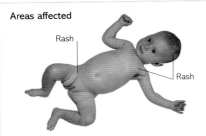

Rash

Rash

✳ Faint red rash over the face, neck, and shoulders, and in the skin creases, such as the elbows, groin, and knees

✳ Flushed and hot appearance

How is it treated?

What should I do first?

1 Check your baby's clothing. She may be wearing too many clothes for the air temperature.

2 Undress your baby and bathe her in tepid water. Gently pat her dry to remove most of the moisture. Allow the rest to evaporate – this will cool her skin down.

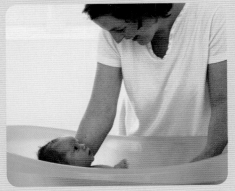

Should I seek medical help?

Consult your doctor only if the rash does not disappear 12 hours after the baby has cooled down.

What might the doctor do?

Your doctor or nurse will examine your baby to exclude any other reason for the rash, and will probably advise you to dress your baby in natural fibres, which do not trap the sweat.

What can I do to help?

✳ Check that the temperature in your baby's room is not too high. Keep the air flowing by opening a window slightly.

✳ Don't overdress your child when the weather is hot.

✳ Don't put wool or synthetic fibres directly against your baby's skin. Dress her in a cotton vest first.

Chapping

Chaps are small cracks in the skin that can be painful if they are deep. In nearly all cases, chapping is preceded by drying out of the skin due to its exposure to cold air or to hot, dry air. Chapping is therefore most common in exposed parts of the body such as on the lips, fingers, hands, and ears.

Possible symptoms

✳ Small cracks in the skin, most commonly on the lips, fingers, hands, and ears

✳ Bleeding, if the cracks are deep

Is it serious?

Chapping is not serious.

How is it treated?

What should I do first?

1 Keep your child's skin well moisturized with cream.

2 Keep him warm in cold weather, particularly his hands and ears.

3 If your child has dry lips, apply lip salve or Vaseline regularly throughout the day.

4 If the chap cracks, place a piece of surgical tape or adhesive tape over it, where possible, for about 12 hours, to stop it drying out and cracking even more. Do not do this to a young baby – he could swallow the tape.

Should I seek medical help?
Consult your doctor if the chaps fail to heal properly, or if they become infected.

What might the doctor do?

✳ Your doctor or nurse may prescribe an emollient cream to keep the skin moist.

✳ If there is an infection, your child may be given antibiotics.

What can I do to help?
Don't wash your child with soap too often during cold weather. Soap removes oil from the skin and makes it rough. An emollient cream or baby lotion can be used instead of soap to clean the skin.

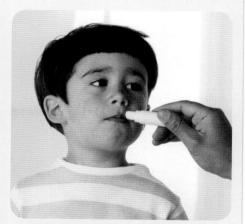

Skin care Keep your child's lips moisturized by using a lip balm, especially during the winter when the skin dries up faster and cracks easily.

SEE ALSO:
CHILBLAINS (p. 46)

Chilblains

Chilblains are areas of red, itchy skin that are the result of hypersensitivity to cold. When the skin of a cold-sensitive child is exposed to cold and damp, the blood vessels beneath the skin close up to conserve heat, causing it to become numb and pale. When the blood vessels dilate again with warmth, the skin becomes red and itchy. Chilblains usually appear on the ankles, hands and feet, and on the back of the legs.

Are they serious?

Chilblains are not serious, but they can be very irritating.

Possible symptoms

* Pale, numb skin, particularly on the hands and feet

* Red, swollen, itchy skin when the area warms up

Common sites

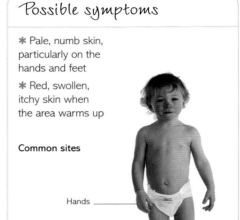

Hands

Back of legs

Feet

How are they treated?

What should I do first?

1 If your child has been out in the cold without sufficient warm clothing and then complains of itchiness, dust the skin with talcum powder or cornflour to ease the irritation.

2 Stop your child from breaking the skin of the affected areas by covering them with clothing, or putting mittens on him.

Should I seek medical help?

Seek medical advice if the chilblains give your child a great deal of discomfort.

What might the doctor do?

Very occasionally a vasodilator cream may be prescribed to improve circulation.

What can I do to help?

* Keep all the susceptible parts on your child's body covered up and warm in damp and cold weather.

* Put thermal insoles in your child's shoes to keep his feet warm.

SEE ALSO:
ITCHING (p. 35)

Boils

A boil is a large, tender, red lump that results when a hair follicle becomes infected with bacteria (*staphylococci*). The pus-filled lump gradually comes to a head and bursts after about two or three days, or it may heal on its own without bursting and slowly disappear. Because the hair follicles are so close together, the bacteria can infect a wide area, causing more boils to occur. This is most likely to happen on the face. The boils usually appear on areas where there are pressure points, such as where a collar rubs, or on the buttocks.

Is it serious?

Although unsightly, a boil is not serious and most boils generally clear up within two weeks. It can, however, be painful, especially if it develops over a bony area such as the jaw, where the skin is stretched tight.

Possible symptoms

* Large, painful, red lump

* Increasing tenderness and throbbing as pus builds up inside the lump. After a day or two, the red lump forms a white or yellow pus-filled centre, which may or may not burst

Cross–section of skin

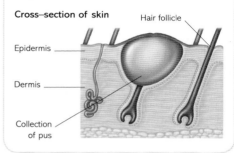

Hair follicle

Epidermis

Dermis

Collection of pus

How are they treated?

What should I do first?
1 Put a sterile gauze dressing over the boil.

2 Do not squeeze the boil, even when it comes to a head. Squeezing will spread the infection to the surrounding area.

Should I seek medical help?
Seek medical advice if the boil does not come to a head within five days or is causing a lot of pain; seek advice as soon as possible if red streaks spread from the centre, as this could mean that the infection is spreading.

What might the doctor do?
* Your doctor or nurse will examine the boil and the surrounding area. If there is pus under the skin, the boil may be lanced and drained.

* If there is an infection, or if your child has had a number of boils over the previous

months, he may be given antibiotic tablets to prevent the spread of the infection.

* If your child is suffering from a crop of boils, your doctor or nurse may prescribe a special antiseptic to put in the bath water.

* If the boils are recurrent, your child will be referred to a dermatologist to find out the underlying cause.

What can I do to help?
* Once the boil has burst, keep it covered to stop your child from scratching the area.

* If the boil is in a place where clothing might rub it, put a thick pad over the dressing to prevent any friction.

* If his boil is on the buttocks and he is still in nappies, leave them off as much as possible.

Cold sores

Cold sores are tiny blisters that form mostly around the nostrils and lips, but sometimes also elsewhere on the face. The blisters break open and weep, then crust over and disappear. Cold sores are caused by a virus (*Herpes simplex*) that lives permanently in the nerve endings of some adults and children. A rise in skin temperature – perhaps caused by a cold, or by going out in the sun – activates the virus. The first attack may take the form of painful mouth ulcers. Subsequent attacks take the form of skin blisters. Most cold sores last for about 10–14 days.

Possible symptoms

✳ Raised red area, usually around the nostrils and lips, which tingles and feels itchy; tiny blisters then form on the spot

✳ Weeping blisters, which then crust over

Are they serious?

Cold sores are not serious unless they occur near the eye, where they may rarely cause an ulcer to form on the front of the eyeball.

How are they treated?

What should I do first?

1 Once blisters have formed, stop your child from touching the affected area. Keep her hands clean.

2 Obtain the cold sore cream aciclovir from your local pharmacy, and use it as instructed.

Should I seek medical help?

Consult your doctor as soon as possible if a cold sore is near your child's eye. Seek medical help if the cold sores become redder and develop pus-filled centres; they will have become infected with bacteria. Ask for your doctor's advice if your child suffers from recurrent cold sores.

What might the doctor do?

✳ If the cold sores are infected, your child will be prescribed an antibiotic to treat the infection.

What can I do to help?

✳ Make sure that your child uses her own towel and face cloth.

✳ Don't let your child kiss anyone, especially other children. The virus can be transmitted from one person to another this way.

✳ If your child tends to develop cold sores after exposure to sunlight, smear a sunblock on her lips or nose when she plays out in the sun.

SEE ALSO:

BLISTERS (p. 41)

MOUTH ULCERS (p. 81)

SUNBURN (p. 43)

Nappy rash

Nappy rash is a skin condition that affects the area normally covered by a baby's nappy, and can occur whether the nappies used are fabric or disposable.

There are several causes of nappy rash, but it is most commonly caused by urine and stools being left in contact with the skin for too long. Bottlefed babies are more likely to suffer from this form of nappy rash than breastfed ones.

Nappy rash can also be caused by not drying your baby thoroughly enough after bathing. In such cases, the nappy rash is usually confined to the skin creases at the top of the thighs. If the rash covers most of the nappy area, and you use fabric nappies, it may be due to an allergic reaction to the chemicals in the washing powder used to wash them, or to a fabric conditioner. This reaction is an early sign of a form of eczema, known as atopic eczema.

Possible symptoms

- ✳ Redness over nappy area
- ✳ Redness that starts around the genitals and is accompanied by a strong smell of ammonia
- ✳ Tight, papery skin with inflamed spots that have pus-filled centres
- ✳ Redness that starts around the anus and moves over the buttocks and on to the thighs

A rash that starts around the anus and moves over the buttocks and on to the thighs may not be nappy rash at all, but a thrush infection.

Is it serious?

Nappy rash is not serious, and can be easily prevented and treated at home.

How is it treated?

What should I do first?

1 If you notice redness on your baby's bottom, wash it with warm water and dry thoroughly. Apply barrier cream to prevent skin irritation.

2 Change nappies and wash your baby's bottom at least every two to three hours, and as soon as she has had a bowel motion. Leave off the nappy whenever possible.

3 Use one-way disposable nappy liners next to her skin, as these let urine pass through to the nappy while remaining dry. Don't use talcum powder at all. It irritates the skin.

4 Check inside her mouth. If there are white patches, try to wipe them off. If they leave raw, red patches, your baby has oral thrush, which may have caused the rash.

Should I seek medical help?

Consult the doctor if these measures fail to clear the rash within a few days, or if you think your baby has thrush.

What might the doctor do?

If the nappy rash has become infected, your doctor may prescribe antibiotics. In case your baby has signs of eczema, your doctor or nurse may advise you to change the brand of washing powder or conditioner you use. If the nappy rash is caused by thrush, your child will be prescribed an anti-fungal cream.

SEE ALSO:

ECZEMA (p. 51)

THRUSH (p. 121)

Cradle cap

Cradle cap is a thick, yellow encrustation on the scalp. It occurs mainly in babies, although children up to the age of three can have cradle cap. The yellow scales appear in small patches, or can cover the entire scalp. Cradle cap is not due to poor hygiene. Babies who suffer from it probably just have greasier scalps.

Possible symptoms

✳ Thick, yellowish scales over part or all of the scalp

Is it serious?

Cradle cap may appear unsightly, but it is quite harmless unless it is accompanied by red, scaly areas elsewhere on your baby's body, in which case your baby may have seborrhoeic eczema.

How is it treated?

What should I do first?

1 Do not try to remove the scales with your fingers. If they won't brush out, they must be loosened first.

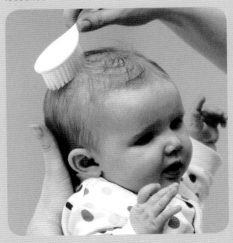

2 Smear a little baby oil or Vaseline on to your baby's scalp and leave overnight. This makes the scales soft and loose, and they will wash away when you shampoo the next day.

3 Do not use anti-dandruff shampoos without consulting your doctor.

Should I seek medical help?

Consult your doctor if you are worried about the condition or if your baby has any red, scaly areas elsewhere.

What might the doctor do?

Your doctor, nurse, or health visitor will recommend a special shampoo to prevent the scales from forming, and give advice on brushing and other home treatments that help prevent cradle cap.

What can I do to help?

✳ You can prevent scales from building up by brushing through your baby's hair daily, even if there is very little of it, with a soft-bristled brush.

✳ Never rub the scalp very hard when washing your child's hair. Shampoos remove dirt within seconds, so you only need to bring the shampoo to a lather and then rinse it off thoroughly.

✳ If the cradle cap becomes quite hard and thick, you may have to continue the baby oil or Vaseline treatment over a 10-day period to loosen all the encrustations.

SEE ALSO:
ECZEMA (p. 51)

Eczema

Eczema is an allergic skin condition which produces an extremely itchy, dry, scaly, red rash on the face, neck, and hands, and in the creases of the limbs.

The most common form of eczema in children is atopic eczema, which usually develops when a baby is about two to three months old, or at around the age of four to five months, when solid foods are first introduced into his diet. Certain foods, most commonly dairy products, eggs, and wheat, and skin irritants such as pet fur, wool, or washing powders, are among the main causes. An attack of eczema can also be triggered by stress, or an emotional upset of any kind. It is quite common for eczema to be followed by other allergic complaints such as hayfever and penicillin sensitivity. It is also common for a child with eczema to suffer from asthma. Although most children grow out of eczema by the age of three, the allergic conditions may remain.

Possible symptoms

* Dry, red, scaly skin, which is extremely itchy. The rash usually starts off as minute pearly blisters beneath the skin's surface
* Sleeplessness if the itchiness is very bad

Another form of eczema, known as seborrhoeic eczema, occurs most commonly on the scalps of young babies (cradle cap), on the eyelashes and eyelids, in the external ear canal (*otitis externa*), and in the greasy areas around the nostrils, ears, and groin. Seborrhoeic eczema is not as itchy as atopic eczema and responds well to treatment.

Is it serious?
Although irritating, eczema is not serious.

How is it treated?

What should I do first?

1 If your child is scratching himself, inspect his neck, scalp, face, hands, and the creases of his elbows, knees, and groin for any rash.

2 Keep his fingernails short to minimize the possibility of breaking the skin. If the skin becomes broken, put mittens or gloves on him to prevent him from scratching the affected area.

3 If you've just started weaning your breastfed child, return to breast feeds until you see your doctor. If you have been using formula milk, return to that.

4 Apply an oily calamine lotion to ease irritation and soothe the skin. Don't apply any astringent lotions.

5 Stop washing your child with soap and water as it removes oils from the skin. Use cleansing creams instead.

6 Put bath oil in his bath water to soothe the skin.

Should I seek medical help?
Seek medical advice if you suspect your child may have eczema.

Continued on page 52

Eczema: continued

What might the doctor do?

✳ Your doctor will ask you about your family's medical history, and in particular whether anyone related to you or your partner has ever suffered from eczema-related conditions, such as asthma or hayfever.

✳ Your doctor will ask you about any changes in your child's diet, whether you have recently changed washing powders, whether you have just brought a pet into the house, and whether your child wears natural or synthetic fibres.

✳ If you have just started weaning your baby from the breast or bottle, your doctor may recommend that you avoid dairy products and continue with breastfeeding or formula milk, or recommend other types of milk instead.

✳ Your doctor may prescribe an anti-inflammatory skin cream to reduce redness, scaliness, and itchiness. In severe cases, steroid creams may be prescribed. These should be used sparingly. Your doctor may also recommend emollient creams or ointments for your child.

✳ Your doctor may prescribe antihistamine medication to help your child go to sleep if the itching is keeping him awake at night.

✳ If your child's skin has become infected through scratching, your doctor may prescribe antibiotics to relieve itching.

✳ Your doctor will advise you to add bath oil to your child's bath water, and to stop using soap as this can be an irritant. The oil will help to keep your child's skin supple and moisturized.

What can I do to help?

✳ Continue to use an emollient cream whenever your child washes. This will keep his skin soft, prevent it from drying out, and will damp down the itchiness as well.

✳ Underplay the condition in front of your child. Your anxiety can make it worse.

✳ Keep your child's fingernails short, and put gloves or mittens on his hands at night so that his scratching doesn't cause the skin to break and become infected.

✳ Make sure all of your child's clothes, and anything else that comes next to his skin, are rinsed thoroughly to remove all traces of any powders and fabric conditioners that could irritate his skin.

✳ You may need to consider finding a new home for your family pet if the reaction is found to be caused by pet fur.

✳ Dress your child with cotton next to his skin at all times.

✳ Remove as many irritants from your child's environment as possible. For example, feather and down pillows can be a source of irritation.

✳ Don't eliminate any foods from your child's diet without your doctors supervision.

Hives

Hives (also called urticaria or nettle rash), is a skin condition. The rash that results is easy to recognize: the skin erupts into white lumps on a red base, known as weals. The weals can be as small as pimples, or may be centimetres across. Hives can be caused by skin contact with an allergen, such as primulas, or it can result from eating certain foods, such as strawberries or shellfish, or from taking certain drugs, particularly penicillin and aspirin. Hives is common after a nettle sting. Each crop of weals is very itchy and lasts up to an hour. It then disappears, to be replaced by more weals elsewhere.

Is it serious?

Hives is not serious, but if it appears on the face, especially in or around the mouth, and is accompanied by swelling, you should dial 999/112 for emergency help. This allergic reaction is known as angioneurotic oedema, and if the swelling spreads to the tongue or the throat, it can cause severe breathing problems.

Possible symptoms

✳ White lumps on a red base

✳ Extremely itchy rash

✳ Weals that disappear within an hour or so to be replaced elsewhere by other weals

✳ Swelling on the face

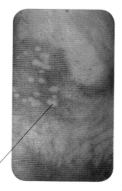

Classic appearance of rash

White lumps

How is it treated?

What should I do first?
1 Apply calamine lotion to the weals to soothe the skin.

2 Give your child a warm bath to relieve his itching.

Should I seek medical help?
Dial 999/112 for emergency help if hives on your child's face cause swelling, particularly in and around the mouth. Check with your doctor or nurse as soon as possible if the weals have not disappeared after several days, or if your child is miserable with the itchiness.

What might the doctor do?
✳ Your doctor may prescribe antihistamine medicine to relieve itchiness.

✳ Your doctor may give your child an injection of adrenalin if the swelling is causing breathing problems.

What can I do to help?
If your child has frequent attacks, make a note of any new foods he might have eaten. Provided it is not an essential food for a growing child, you can exclude it for a week or two, then reintroduce it and watch for a reaction.

SEE ALSO:
ITCHING (p. 35)

Athlete's foot

This is a fungal infection that affects the soft area between and underneath the toes. At an advanced stage, it also affects the nails. It is contagious, and is usually picked up by walking barefoot in communal areas, such as shower rooms, gyms, and swimming pools. The infection is aggravated by sweaty feet, because the fungus tinea, which also causes ringworm elsewhere on the body, thrives in warm and moist conditions.

Is it serious?

Athlete's foot is a common condition, requiring simple treatment and good hygiene to cure it. However, as it is contagious, you should act promptly so that the infection does not spread.

Possible symptoms

* ✳ Blistered skin between the toes, which, when scratched leaves raw skin underneath
* ✳ Dry, peeling skin
* ✳ Thick, yellow toenails

Possible sites of blistered skin

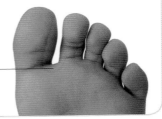

Vulnerable areas between the toes

How is it treated?

What should I do first?

1 If your child has itchy feet, carefully check the area between his toes and underneath them for any white blisters and redness.

2 Also check underneath the foot for blisters.

3 Check the condition of your child's toenails.

4 Buy an antifungal foot powder or cream from your local pharmacy, and after washing and drying the feet thoroughly, apply the treatment, following the manufacturer's instructions.

5 Emphasize to your child that he must not go barefoot until the condition has cleared up.

6 Keep your child's towel and bath mat separate from those of the rest of the family, and wash them every day.

Should I seek medical help?

Seek medical help if the underside of the foot is affected, or the nails are yellowing. Consult your doctor if home measures fail to improve the condition within two or three weeks.

What might the doctor do?

* ✳ If the fungus has affected the toenails, your doctor will prescribe an antifungal medication that may need to be taken for as long as nine months.

* ✳ If your home measures have failed, your doctor will prescribe another antifungal powder or cream.

What can I do to help?

* ✳ Make sure your child wears clean socks every day, preferably cotton or wool.

* ✳ Rotate your child's shoes so that he does not wear the same pair all the time.

SEE ALSO:
RINGWORM (p. 56)

Impetigo

Impetigo is a bacterial skin infection that is most often seen around the lips, nose, and ears. It is caused by very common skin organisms (*staphylococcus* and *streptococcus*), which are carried in the nose and on the skin. The rash starts as small blisters, which break and then crust over to become yellow-brown scabs. The condition is most often seen in school-age children, and is very contagious.

Is it serious?

Impetigo rarely has serious effects, but because it is highly contagious it should be treated as soon as possible.

Possible symptoms

* Tiny blisters around the nose and mouth or ears, which ooze and harden to form crusty, yellow-brown scabs

How is it treated?

What should I do first?

1 If the rash on your child's face starts to weep, stop him from touching it. Gently wash away any crusts with warm water, and pat his face dry with a paper towel. Make sure that your child's facecloth and towel are kept separate from those of the rest of the family to avoid spreading the infection.

2 Don't send your child to school until you have visited the doctor and confirmed the diagnosis.

Should I seek medical help?

Seek medical advice as soon as possible if you suspect impetigo.

What might the doctor do?

* If there are only a few blisters, your doctor will prescribe an antibiotic cream, which should clear up the impetigo within five days.

* If there are a lot of blisters, your doctor might prescribe a course of antibiotics to be taken by mouth to eradicate the infection from your child's body.

What can I do to help?

* Before applying the ointment, wash away any yellow crusts with warm water, and pat dry with a paper towel.

* Be meticulous about hygiene. Wash your hands before and after administering the treatment, and encourage your child to keep his hands away from his face. Keep his fingernails short to reduce the risk of spreading the infection to other parts of the body.

* Be very strict with your child if he sucks his thumb, bites his nails, or picks his nose. This can spread the infection.

* When the infection has cleared, keep the affected area moist with emollient cream.

SEE ALSO:
BLISTERS (p. 41)

Ringworm

Ringworm is a fungal infection of the skin and hair that shows itself in the form of bald patches in the hair, and as round, reddish, or grey scaly patches on the skin. As the infection spreads, the edges of the ring remain scaly, while the centre begins to look more like normal skin. Ringworm is usually contracted from animals, such as household pets, or from other infected humans.

Is it serious?
Although not a serious disorder, ringworm is irritating and looks very unattractive. Ringworm is also highly contagious, and must therefore be treated promptly.

Possible symptoms

✳ Red or grey scaly rings on any part of the body, particularly warm, moist areas, and on the scalp, where they produce bald patches

✳ Itchiness in the ringed areas

How is it treated?

What should I do first?
1 If your child is scratching, check all over her body for the distinctive rings of ringworm.

2 Do not try to treat it yourself. Wash your hands after examining your child. Discourage her from touching the infected areas.

3 Keep your child away from school until you have visited the doctor.

Should I seek medical help?
Seek medical advice as ringworm is contagious, as well as irritating for your child.

What might the doctor do?
Your doctor will prescribe an antifungal cream for the skin, and antibiotic tablets for the scalp. The tablets will have to be taken for at least four weeks.

What can I do to help?
✳ Throw away any brushes, combs, or headgear your child may have used while infected. Disinfectant will not destroy the fungus.

✳ Keep your child's face cloth and towel separate from those of the rest of the family to avoid spreading the infection through the household.

✳ Always make sure that you and your child wash your hands thoroughly both before and after touching the affected areas.

✳ If you think that your pet is a possible source of ringworm, take it to the vet as soon as possible.

✳ Ringworm on the skin clears up quickly, but treatment of the scalp could take a couple of weeks or more to get better. Get your child some form of headgear to hide the bald patches if she is bothered by them.

SEE ALSO:
ITCHING (p. 35)

Lice (nits)

The head louse is a tiny insect that infests the hair on the human head. The adult louse lays its eggs (nits) at the root of the hair, to which they become firmly attached. This distinguishes them from dandruff, which can be flaked off easily with a fingernail. The eggs hatch after two weeks, and the lice bite the scalp to suck blood. Your child's head will be itchy where the lice bite, particularly after strenuous exercise, when she is hot. Your child can become infested by contact with another infested child or adult, particularly after she begins school and if she shares her hats or combs.

Are they serious?
Lice and nits are irritating, but they can be easily eradicated, and are not serious.

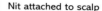

Possible symptoms

* Itchy scalp, particularly when the head is hot

* Tiny, pearly white eggs covering the roots of the hair

Nit attached to scalp   **Adult louse**

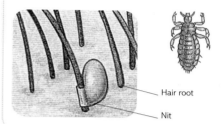

Hair root

Nit

How are they treated?

What should I do first?
1 If your child scratches, inspect the roots of the hair for nits.

2 If you find them, keep your child away from school or nursery, and administer anti-lice shampoo as per the manufacturer's instructions. Inform the school or nursery.

3 First wash her hair thoroughly, then soak it in plenty of shampoo and comb through with a nit comb.

4 If you find lice or nits, repeat this process four times over the next two weeks.

5 Examine the heads of the rest of your family for nits, and treat in the same way. If anyone in your family has been in contact with someone who has lice, it is quite likely that the insects have transferred from one head to another.

Should I seek medical help?
Check with your doctor or nurse as soon as possible if the treatment doesn't work, or if you are not sure that your child has head lice.

What might the doctor do?
* Your doctor or nurse will ask you about the self-help treatment you have used.

What can I do to help?
* Clean your child's headgear, brush, and combs thoroughly.

* If your child starts scratching again, repeat the treatment.

* Check your child's head every two to three weeks.

Scabies

Scabies is an irritating, itchy rash caused by a tiny mite. The burrowing and egg-laying of these mites produce a rash that nearly always affects the hands and fingers, particularly the clefts between the fingers. It may also affect the ankles, feet, toes, elbows, and the area around the genitals. The symptoms of scabies may take up to six weeks to appear. When the eggs hatch, they are easily passed on from one person to another by direct contact. They can also be picked up from bedding or linen that is infested with the mites.

Is it serious?

Scabies is not serious, but it is contagious, and can run through a family or a school class if not treated promptly.

Possible symptoms

✳ Intense itchiness

✳ Fine, short lines that end in a black spot the size of a pinhead, most often found between the fingers

✳ Scabs on the itchy areas

Common site of rash

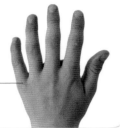

Typical site of
scabies rash _____

How is it treated?

What should I do first?

1 If your child is scratching a lot, look for the fine lines of the mites' burrows.

2 If you suspect scabies, keep your child away from school until you have administered the treatment.

3 Try to discourage her from scratching. This may hinder the doctor's diagnosis, and cause sores to form that could become infected.

Should I seek medical help?

Seek medical advice if you suspect scabies, or if your child is scratching a lot.

What might the doctor do?

✳ Your doctor or nurse will prescribe a lotion to be applied in sufficient quantity for the whole family to be treated.

What can I do to help?

✳ After thorough washing, apply the lotion that your doctor has prescribed on the whole body below the neck, and leave to dry. Don't wash it off for at least 24 hours. To ensure that you have completely cleared the mites, repeat the procedure for a further 24 hours in a day or two.

✳ Carry out the treatment for other members of the family simultaneously.

✳ Launder or air all bedding and clothing to eradicate the mite. It does not live for longer than five or six days after it is removed from human skin.

SEE ALSO:
ITCHING (p. 35)

Ingrowing toenails

When a toenail fails to grow straight out from the nailbed, but instead curves over into the sides of the toe, it is referred to as an ingrowing toenail. This occurs most often on the nail of the big toe, and causes pain and discomfort. An ingrowing toenail is more likely to occur if the toe is broad and plump, if the toenail is cut down at the sides instead of straight across, if it is small, or if tight shoes and socks have pushed the nail into the skin. If left untreated, the nail will penetrate the skin, possibly becoming infected, causing painful inflammation and a discharge of pus around the edges of the nail.

Are they serious?

An ingrowing toenail can be very painful, but it is not usually serious.

How are they treated?

What should I do first?
1 Examine the skin around the nail to see if the nail has penetrated the skin.

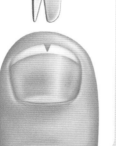

2 Cut a tiny V shape in the top edge of the nail to relieve pressure on the sides of the nail.

3 If there is any sign of redness or pus, apply a sterile dressing to the toe.

Should I seek medical help?
Seek medical advice if the nail has penetrated the skin, if you notice any redness or pus around your child's toenail, or if ingrowing toenails are a recurrent problem.

What might the doctor do?
* Your child may be prescribed antibiotic tablets to clear up the infection.

* If the problem seems to be recurrent, you may have to consult a surgeon, who will examine your child's toe and see whether the ingrowing edge of the toenail should be removed. This is not a serious operation.

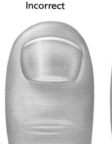

Incorrect

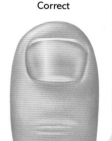

Correct

What can I do to help?
* Whenever you cut your child's toenails, trim them straight across, and not too short. Also, cut them regularly.

* Make sure her shoes and socks are not too tight; allow her space to wriggle her toes.

* If her toenail becomes infected, don't put socks on her; cut the toe out of an old shoe, or let her wear sandals while the infection is clearing up.

Verruca

A verruca is a wart on the sole of the foot that has been pushed back into the foot by the pressure of walking. It is highly infectious, and is spread by direct contact with surfaces where people with infected feet have been going barefoot, such as communal swimming pools, showers, and gyms. It takes about two years for the body to build up resistance to the wart virus (after which the warts usually disappear naturally), but because a verruca is painful, and can be spread easily, treatment is always advisable.

Is it serious?

A verruca is never serious, but it can cause pain and discomfort, depending on where it appears on the sole of the foot.

Possible symptoms

✳ Flat white or brown lump on the sole of the foot

✳ Pain in the foot when walking or standing

Common site of verruca

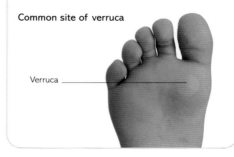

Verruca

How is it treated?

What should I do first?

1 Wash your child's feet and leave them to soak in warm water to soften the skin.

2 With a clean scalpel (available from the chemist), pare away thin layers of the softened verruca very gently. It is always wiser to take off too little rather than draw blood.

3 Apply a proprietary brand of wart treatment, obtainable from a chemist. Don't apply the treatment to healthy skin. To avoid this, use a corn plaster, with a hole the size of the verruca cut out of it, to protect the surrounding areas. After applying the lotion, cover the verruca with a sterile dressing and plaster.

4 Repeat the procedure every day until the verruca has disappeared.

Should I seek medical help?

Seek medical advice immediately if the verruca is painful, if the verrucas are increasing in number, or if home treatment fails.

What might the doctor do?

Your doctor may refer you to a special wart clinic under the supervision of a dermatologist. The verruca will be removed either by treatment with a freezing agent, such as liquid nitrogen, or by being burned off or scraped out under a local anaesthetic.

What can I do to help?

✳ Cover the verruca completely with a secure plaster whenever your child goes barefoot; this should prevent the virus from spreading.

✳ Discourage your child from scratching the verruca. There is a risk he could infect himself elsewhere.

Chapter 4

Eyes, ears, nose, throat, and mouth

Young children are **particularly susceptible** to infections of the eyes, ears, nose, throat, and mouth. This chapter will give you practical advice on **how to protect your child** and help him **recover.**

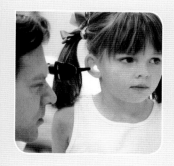
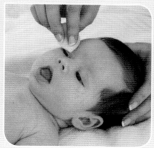
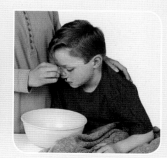

Diagnosis guide

To use this section, look for the symptom most similar to the one your child is suffering from, then turn to the relevant entry. See also p. 13 for a list of symptoms requiring emergency treatment.

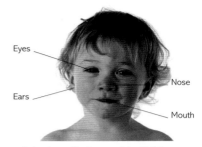

Eyes

Nose

Ears

Mouth

Eyes

✶ Sore, watery eye, possibly **Conjunctivitis**, see p. 77, or **Foreign object in eye**, see p. 78. If accompanied by sneezing, possibly **Hayfever**, see p. 89

✶ Pain underneath the eyes, possibly **Sinusitis**, see p. 65

✶ Swollen, red area on the eyelid, possibly **Styes**, see p. 75

✶ Pus oozing from the inner corner of the eye, possibly **Sticky eye**, see p. 76

Ears

✶ Pain in and around the ear, possibly **Toothache**, see p. 80, or **Earache**, see p. 70, or **Otitis externa**, see p. 71

✶ Impaired hearing with fullness in the ear, possibly **Glue ear**, see p. 69, or **Foreign object in ear**, see p. 72

✶ Pain inside the ear canal made worse when the earlobe is pulled, possibly **Otitis externa**, see p. 71

Nose

✶ Bleeding nose, possibly **Nosebleed**, see p. 74, or **Foreign object in nose**, see p. 73

Mouth

✶ Red or white sore, ulcerated area inside the mouth, possibly **Mouth ulcers**, see p. 81

✶ Yellow or white frothy patches in the mouth, possibly oral **Thrush**, see p. 121

✶ Desire to bite on any hard object accompanied by irritability and a swollen area on the gum in a young baby, possibly **Teething**, see p. 79

✶ Red, inflamed lump on the gum sometimes with swollen glands, possibly **Dental abscess**, see p. 82, or in a young baby, **Teething**, see p. 79

Cold and allergy symptoms

Swollen neck glands
accompanied by a fever, possibly **Sore throat**, see p. 66, **Tonsillitis**, see p. 67, or **Laryngitis**, see p. 68

Hoarse cough or loss of voice,
possibly **Croup**, see p. 88, or **Laryngitis**, see p. 68

Sneezing, with a runny nose
and itchy eyes, possibly **Hayfever**, see p. 89

Diarrhoea, vomiting, or nausea
accompanied by shivering, fever, and a cough, possibly **Influenza**, see p. 87

Runny nose
often with a sore throat and fever, possibly **Common cold**, see p. 63, or **Influenza**, see p. 87

Runny nose with a clear discharge
and coughing, especially at night, possibly **Catarrh**, see p. 64, or **Common cold**, see p. 63

Common cold

The common cold is caused by a virus that enters the body through the nasal passages and throat, and causes inflammation of the mucous membranes lining these passages. The body's defences take around 10 days to fight off the virus.

Is it serious?

A common cold is not serious. However, because it lowers the body's resistance, complications such as bronchitis can sometimes arise. A cold should be regarded more seriously in a baby because minor symptoms, such as a blocked nose, can cause feeding problems.

Possible symptoms

* Sneezing
* Runny or blocked nose
* Raised temperature
* Coughing
* Sore throat
* Aching muscles
* Irritability
* Catarrh

How is it treated?

What should I do first?

1 Take your child's temperature. If it is high (37°C (98.6°F) or more), put her to bed and bring her temperature down (see p. 15).

2 Check your child's nasal discharge. Yellow discharge can indicate a secondary infection, while clear mucus could signify hayfever.

3 Don't give any shop-bought medicines without your doctor's advice.

Should I seek medical help?

Consult your doctor immediately if you think your child has developed a secondary infection. If your baby is having trouble sleeping or feeding, consult your doctor or health visitor immediately, too.

What might the doctor do?

* Your doctor or nurse will treat a secondary infection to the cold.

* Nose drops may be prescribed to make feeding easier. Use as directed, as over-use can damage the nose lining.

What can I do to help?

* Ease your baby's breathing by placing a pillow under the mattress to raise her head.

* Give your child plenty to drink and teach her to blow her nose by blowing one nostril at a time.

* If possible, create a humid atmosphere in your child's bedroom.

* Smear Vaseline on to your child's nose and upper lip if they are sore.

* A hot bedtime drink of fresh lemon juice and water will soothe her sore throat, and clear her nasal passages.

SEE ALSO:

BRONCHITIS (p. 86)

CATARRH (p. 64)

CROUP (p. 88)

HAYFEVER (p. 89)

SORE THROAT (p. 66)

Catarrh

Catarrh is an excess of mucus in the nose and throat. It may be the result of a common cold, or it may be a symptom of influenza. One of the most severe forms of acute catarrh occurs in hayfever, when the allergic reaction of a runny nose is accompanied by itchy, tearful eyes, and sneezing.

Chronic catarrh is usually caused by sinusitis. The mucus from the infected sinuses runs down the back of the throat, causing the child to cough, particularly when he is lying down. Breathing becomes difficult, and if a great deal of mucus is swallowed, this unpleasant sensation could lead to vomiting. Occasionally, the symptoms of catarrh may also indicate a middle ear infection, enlarged adenoids, or nasal polyps.

Possible symptoms

- ✳ Nasal congestion
- ✳ Runny nose with a clear discharge
- ✳ Coughing, especially at night
- ✳ Difficulty in feeding in small babies
- ✳ Vomiting if the mucus is swallowed

Is it serious?

Catarrh, with a minor illness, is not serious. However, chronic catarrh will require treatment.

How is it treated?

What should I do first?

1 Encourage your child to blow his nose frequently. The catarrh will probably not need any more treatment than this.

2 If your child is coughing at night, prop him up with pillows, or raise the height of the cot – a thick book under the mattress by his head would be about the right elevation – so that the mucus doesn't drip down his throat.

3 Never use nose drops without seeking medical advice.

Should I seek medical help?

Seek medical advice as soon as possible if the catarrh is making feeding difficult for your baby. Consult your doctor if you think the catarrh may be an allergic reaction, such as hayfever, or if it persists for no apparent reason.

What might the doctor do?

✳ For a baby, nose drops may be prescribed to relieve the congestion.

✳ If your doctor thinks it is caused by an allergy, he will examine for possible causes.

✳ If the catarrh is caused by chronic sinusitis or a middle ear infection, antibiotics will be prescribed. If it is caused by enlarged adenoids or nasal polyps, surgical removal may be recommended.

What can I do to help?

Teach your child to blow his nose by clearing one nostril at a time.

SEE ALSO:

COMMON COLD (p. 63)

HAYFEVER (p. 89)

INFLUENZA (p. 87)

SINUSITIS (p. 65)

Sinusitis

Sinusitis is a bacterial infection of the cheek (maxillary) and forehead (frontal) sinuses. These air-filled spaces, grouped around the eyes and nose, make the skull bones light, and give the voice resonance. Infections of the sinuses are rare in babies because their sinuses are not fully developed, but in older children some degree of sinusitis often accompanies a common cold, cough, or sore throat.

A yellow-green discharge of pus from the nose is often the sign that your child has sinusitis.

Is it serious?

Sinusitis is not a serious ailment, although it can become chronic if it is not treated effectively when it appears; so consult a doctor as soon as the first symptoms appear.

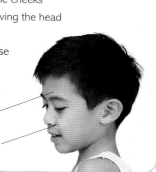

Possible symptoms

* Yellow-green discharge of pus from the nose where previously there was a clear, runny discharge
* Pain over the cheeks
* Pain on moving the head
* Slight fever
* Blocked nose

Affected areas

Frontal sinuses

Maxillary sinuses

How is it treated?

What should I do first?
1 If your child has a cold, cough, or sore throat, watch out for a change in the colour of his nasal discharge.

2 Check to see if there is a foreign object lodged in your child's nose. The discharge will then be foul-smelling and stained with blood. Seek medical help immediately if you cannot easily remove the foreign body.

3 If there is no foreign object, relieve his blocked nose by encouraging him, if he is old enough (older than 10), to blow his nose regularly.

Should I seek medical help?
Seek medical advice if the yellow-green nasal discharge continues for more than two days.

What might the doctor do?
* Your doctor will prescribe antibiotics to eradicate the infection.

* If sinusitis is recurrent, your doctor will refer your child to an ear, nose, and throat specialist to see whether surgical draining of the sinuses is necessary.

What can I do to help?
* If your child complains of a headache or fever, give him liquid paracetamol or ibuprofen.

* Don't overheat your child's bedroom. Keep the air cool and humid; a dry atmosphere makes the symptoms worse.

SEE ALSO:
COMMON COLD (p. 63)
COUGH (p. 85)
FOREIGN OBJECT IN NOSE (p. 73)
SORE THROAT (p. 66)

Sore throat

A sore throat is usually a symptom of an infection of the respiratory tract. While a baby or young child may not be able to tell you about the raw feeling in his throat, you will notice that he has difficulty swallowing. Sore throats can occur because of inflammation of the tonsils (tonsillitis), caused by the *streptococcus* bacterium, or more usually by a virus, such as the common cold or influenza. If there is inflammation elsewhere, as there is in the larynx when your child has laryngitis, this can also give a raw feeling in the throat.

Is it serious?

Most sore throats are not serious. However, if your child is allergic to the *streptococcus* bacterium and he has a streptococcal infection in the throat, this could have effects elsewhere in his body. Occasional more serious complications that can occur include illnesses such as nephritis and rheumatic fever.

How is it treated?

What should I do first?

1 If your child complains of a sore throat, or if he is having difficulty swallowing and is off his food, carefully examine his throat in a good light, with his head held back and the tongue depressed gently with the handle of a clean spoon. Ask him to say a long "aaah". This will open up the throat wide enough so that you will be able to check to see if there is any inflammation, or if the tonsils are enlarged.

2 Gently run your fingers down either side of your child's neck and under his chin to check if he has any swelling in the glands – they will feel like large peas under the skin (see p. 67).

3 Take your child's temperature to see if he has a fever.

4 As the sore throat is most likely to be caused by some sort of infection, keep your child away from school or nursery school until you have had medical advice and obtained confirmation that the problem is not contagious.

Should I seek medical help?

Seek medical advice as soon as possible, as a sore throat will cause your child discomfort.

Streptococcal infection of the throat should be treated promptly to avoid complications.

What might the doctor do?

Your doctor will examine your child to determine the cause of the sore throat. If it is a *streptococcus* bacterium, your doctor will prescribe antibiotics.

What can I do to help?

✳ Soothe your child's sore throat with cold drinks or hot lemon drinks.

✳ Give your child plenty of liquids. If he isn't eating because it hurts to swallow, liquidize foods where possible. You can also offer him soups, yogurt, and smoothies.

SEE ALSO:

COMMON COLD (p. 63)
FEVER (p. 26)
INFLUENZA (p. 87)
LARYNGITIS (p. 68)
MUMPS (p. 29)
TONSILLITIS (p. 67)

Tonsillitis

Positioned at the back of the throat, the tonsils are the body's first line of defence. They trap and kill bacteria, preventing them from entering the respiratory tract. In the process, they can become infected, causing tonsillitis. The adenoids, at the back of the nose, are usually affected as well.

Babies under the age of about one rarely suffer from tonsillitis; it occurs mainly among school-age children, when the relatively large tonsils and adenoids are exposed to infectious microbes. As resistance to infectious microbes increases, attacks should lessen.

Is it serious?

Tonsillitis is not serious unless repeatedly accompanied by infection of the middle ear, which could lead to hearing problems.

Possible symptoms

* Sore throat, possibly bad enough to cause difficulty in swallowing

* Red and enlarged tonsils, possibly covered in yellow spots

* Mouth-breathing, snoring, and a nasal voice

* Swollen glands in the neck

* Unpleasant breath

* A fever

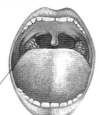

Affected area

Enlarged tonsils

How is it treated?

What should I do first?

1 If your child has a sore throat or difficulty eating, check his throat. Ask him to say a long "aaah". You should be able to see if his tonsils are red, enlarged, or covered with spots.

2 Take your child's temperature to see if he has a fever, and check if his glands are swollen – they will feel like large peas under the skin.

3 Ask him if he has an earache. In a young child, note whether he pulls or rubs his ears. Check to see if there is any discharge.

Should I seek medical help?

Seek medical advice as soon as possible if you suspect tonsillitis.

What might the doctor do?

* Your doctor may take a throat swab to identify the infection, and will prescribe antibiotics for bacterial tonsillitis.

* Your doctor will examine your child's ears, and if there are any signs of infection, he will prescribe antibiotics.

* If your child suffers from frequent attacks of tonsillitis, or if enlarged adenoids cause recurrent middle-ear infections, you may be referred to a specialist.

What can I do to help?

* Treat your child as you would for fever.

* Keep his fluid intake up with regular drinks.

* Never give your child a gargle for a sore throat. It can spread infection from the throat to the middle ear.

* Offer him foods that slip down easily, but don't force him to eat.

SEE ALSO:
EARACHE (p. 70), **FEVER** (p. 26), **SORE THROAT** (p. 66)

Laryngitis

Laryngitis is an inflammation of the larynx or the voice box. Many minor viruses, and occasionally bacteria, can enter the body through the throat and quickly infect the larynx. The most obvious symptoms of laryngitis are hoarseness and a dry cough, and sometimes a fever.

Is it serious?

Laryngitis is rarely serious and lasts for less than seven days, even if it is part of a more serious infection, such as tonsillitis or bronchitis. However, in young children, a swollen larynx can obstruct the passage of air, causing breathing difficulties and croup. If laryngitis develops into croup, you should seek medical help.

Possible symptoms

* ✳ Hoarseness or loss of voice
* ✳ Dry cough
* ✳ Slight fever
* ✳ Sore throat
* ✳ Croup, a type of barking cough

Cross-section of the throat

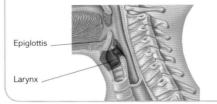

Epiglottis

Larynx

How is it treated?

What should I do first?

1 If the hoarseness is not accompanied by any other symptoms of a respiratory tract infection, such as bronchitis, keep a check on your child's temperature. If it rises above 37°C (98.6°F), there may be another infection.

2 Listen closely for the barking cough of croup.

3 Keep the air in your child's room moist if possible. Open a window to allow air to circulate. This is an effective atmosphere for suppressing a dry cough.

Should I seek medical help?

Seek medical advice as soon as possible if you think your child has croup. Check with your doctor as soon as possible if your child has a fever, or you think he has contracted another infection.

What might the doctor do?

If there is a bacterial infection, such as bronchitis or tonsillitis, your doctor will prescribe antibiotics.

What can I do to help?

✳ Discourage your child from talking out loud. You could make a game of it, and have the whole family talking in whispers.

✳ Give your child plenty of warm drinks to soothe his throat. Try hot lemon and honey, or heat any fruit juice by diluting it with hot water.

SEE ALSO:
BRONCHITIS (p. 86)
COUGH (p. 85)
CROUP (p. 88)
FEVER (p. 26)
TONSILLITIS (p. 67)

Glue ear

Glue ear is a condition that results when the Eustachian tube and middle ear are filled with fluid as a result of infection. The Eustachian tube, which runs from the throat to the ear, produces large quantities of fluid as a response to chronic infections, such as sinusitis, tonsillitis, or, most commonly, infection of the middle ear. If the tube in either ear is blocked by inflammation, the fluid cannot drain and becomes glue-like, impeding the efficient vibration of sound, causing loss of hearing.

Is it serious?

Glue ear should be treated seriously because it can lead to permanent loss of hearing in the affected ear, and can cause problems with speech development and learning.

Possible symptoms

* A feeling of fullness in the ear
* Partial loss of hearing, or deafness in one or both ears

Position of grommet

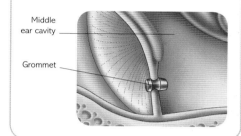

Middle ear cavity

Grommet

How is it treated?

What should I do first?

If your child seems inattentive, and has recently had a cold, do a hearing test. Call out his name softly when his head is averted and see if there is a response. Even if he can hear you, hearing may be impaired in such a way that he cannot tell where you are calling from.

Should I seek medical help?

Seek medical advice as soon as possible if your child's hearing is impaired.

What might the doctor do?

* Your doctor will examine your child's ears with a special instrument called an otoscope.

* Antibiotics may be prescribed to clear up the infection.

* In severe and recurrent cases, your child will probably be referred to an ear, nose, and throat specialist for a hearing test. He may be admitted to a hospital to have the fluid drained off under a general anaesthetic, and grommets may be inserted into the eardrum. These are tiny plastic tubes that allow mucus to drain away. They either fall out after several months, when the ears are healthy again, or can be removed by the specialist. If glue ear is a result of repeated infections or enlarged adenoids, the underlying problem will also be treated to prevent recurrences.

What can I do to help?

* If your child has had grommets inserted, he must always wear a bathing cap when swimming, and should not dive. Most doctors advise against swimming at all with grommets.

* Try to keep the ear as dry as possible.

SEE ALSO:
COMMON COLD (p. 63)
SINUSITIS (p. 65)
TONSILLITIS (p. 67)

Earache

There are a number of causes of earache. The most common is otitis media – an infection of the middle ear. Children under six are more prone to this infection, because the tube that runs from the throat to the ear – the Eustachian tube – is relatively short, and so infections of the nose and throat can easily spread to their middle ear cavity. A child may complain of an earache if he is suffering from toothache or tonsillitis, if the glands in his neck are swollen, or if he has been out in the cold without a hat. Earache with an intense pain may result from otitis externa – an infection of the outer ear – if, for example, a foreign object has been poked into the ear or if a boil has developed.

Possible symptoms

* ✳ Pain in the area around the ear
* ✳ A temperature of over 37°C (98.6°F)
* ✳ Discharge of pus from the ear
* ✳ Deafness
* ✳ Inflammation of the tonsils
* ✳ Pain when the ear is touched
* ✳ Swollen glands
* ✳ Rubbing of the ear in a young child

Is it serious?

Earache with loss of hearing is serious.

How is it treated?

What should I do first?

1 Take your child's temperature to see if he has a fever.

2 Check if there is any discharge from the ear, and whether your child's hearing is diminished. To do this, call his name quietly when his head is averted. See if he turns around.

3 Examine the back of your child's throat to see if the tonsils are abnormally enlarged or red.

4 Check if your child has any inflammation in the outer ear cavity. Don't put a cotton-wool swab into the ear or use eardrops unless your doctor advises it.

Should I seek medical help?

Seek medical advice if your child complains of an earache, as most earache is caused by an infection. Consult a doctor immediately if your child is in pain, has a high fever, or if you notice any discharge from his ear.

Consult a doctor as soon as possible if he is too young to tell you, and is crying, and pulling or rubbing his ear.

What might the doctor do?

Your doctor will examine your child to determine the cause of the earache. If it is caused by a bacterial infection, he will prescribe antibiotics.

What can I do to help?

✳ Place a hot water bottle, covered by a towel, next to your child's ear, and give him paracetamol or ibuprofen to relieve the pain.

✳ Prevent water from entering your child's ear while bathing him.

SEE ALSO:

BOILS (p. 47)

FOREIGN OBJECT IN EAR (p. 72)

MUMPS (p. 29)

OTITIS EXTERNA (p. 71)

TONSILLITIS (p. 67)

TOOTHACHE (p. 80)

Otitis externa

Otitis externa is an infection of the external ear canal – the passage that leads from the ear flap (pinna) to the eardrum. The infection may be caused by a foreign object in the ear, by a boil in the canal, or as the result of damage to the skin from vigorous cleaning or scratching. The infection is more common in children who swim a great deal.

Is it serious?

As the external ear canal does not contain the ear's delicate hearing mechanisms, the infection itself is relatively minor. However, it will always be treated seriously, because in rare cases the infection could spread to the skull bones, and possibly to the brain. Any discharge from the ear should be treated promptly as this could be a symptom of a serious middle ear infection.

Possible symptoms

* Earache
* Redness and tenderness of the ear flap and external ear canal
* Pus-filled boil in the canal
* Discharge from the ear
* Itchy, dry, scaly ear

How is it treated?

What should I do first?

1 Look into the ear canal to check for signs of infection or foreign objects. Remove objects only if you can do so easily. Don't push or poke anything into your child's ear, and discourage him from touching or scratching it.

2 Ask your child to open his mouth wide to see if this causes pain.

3 Pull back gently on the ear flap to see if this causes pain. Clean away any discharge with warm water, soap, and a flannel.

4 Give your child paracetamol or ibuprofen to relieve pain, and place a cotton-wool pad over the ear to absorb any discharge.

Should I seek medical help?

Seek medical advice if you notice any discharge from your child's ear, or if you suspect infection.

What might the doctor do?

* Your doctor will examine your child's ear with an instrument called an otoscope, and may clean out the ear with a probe. Antibiotic eardrops may be prescribed to clear up the infection.

* If there is a foreign object in your child's ear, your doctor will remove it, or refer him to a hospital for its removal.

* If the pain is the result of a boil, your doctor may lance the boil and drain the pus away.

What can I do to help?

* If your child is in pain, give him paracetamol or ibuprofen.

* Prevent water from entering the ear until the infection has cleared completely.

* Never poke cotton-wool swabs into your child's ear to clear wax. They will only push it further into the canal or damage the lining.

* Never use eardrops unless your doctor advises them.

SEE ALSO:

BOILS (p. 47) **EARACHE** (p. 70)

FOREIGN OBJECT IN EAR (p. 72)

Foreign object in ear

The most common foreign objects that get stuck in a child's ear are small items, such as beads, pushed in by the child or by a playmate. Very rarely, a small insect may fly into the ear and be trapped there.

Is it serious?

Any foreign object in the ear that cannot be removed easily should be regarded as serious because it may cause an infection of the external ear canal, otitis externa, or damage the eardrum.

Possible symptoms

✳ Pain and tenderness in the ear
✳ A visible embedded object

How is it treated?

What should I do first?
1 If the object is small and soft, try to remove it with tweezers. If you can't grasp it easily, leave it and seek medical advice as soon as possible.

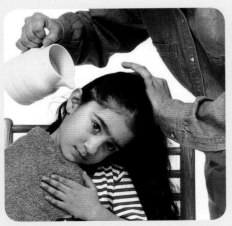

2 If the foreign object is an insect, lay your child on her side or tilt her head to one side with the affected ear uppermost, and pour warm water into the ear. The insect should float out.

Should I get medical help?
Seek medical advice as soon as possible if the object cannot be removed, or if your child complains of pain and tenderness in the ear.

What might the doctor do?
After examining your child's external ear canal, your doctor will remove the object and will treat any damage to the skin, or any infection that may have been caused by the foreign object.

What can I do to help?
Don't let a child under three play with small objects that she could poke into her ear – or into her nose or mouth.

SEE ALSO:
OTITIS EXTERNA (p. 71)

Foreign object in nose

If there is a foreign object of any sort in your child's nose it is most likely to have been pushed in there by your child or a playmate. The problem may not even be noticed by you or your child at first, but after two or three days there will probably be a nosebleed, or perhaps even a blood-stained, foul-smelling discharge from the affected nostril.

Is it serious?

If the foreign object cannot be easily removed from your child's nose, on no account attempt to remove it yourself – you might push it further in. Instead, you should take your child to your nearest hospital emergency department. If the foreign object can be easily removed it is not serious and should have no after-effects. It is more serious if your child inhales the object into her lungs, as this may partially block her air passages and result in breathing difficulties or choking.

How is it treated?

What should I do first?

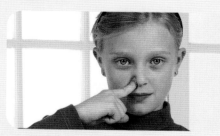

1 If your child is old enough to understand, ask her to hold a finger against the good nostril and blow the affected one to dislodge the foreign object. Don't ask a young child to do this – she might sniff the object back into her air passages.

2 Alternatively, lay your child on her back and shine a light on her face. If you can see the object near the entrance to the nose, and if it is soft, remove it with tweezers. If it is further up the nostril, leave it alone. If your child has breathing problems, treat this as an emergency. Dial 999/112 for emergency help.

Should I seek medical help?
Seek medical advice as soon as possible or take your child to the nearest hospital emergency department if you cannot easily remove the object from her nose.

What might the doctor do?
Your doctor will remove the foreign object with a pair of forceps. If your child is very young, or refuses to stay still, she may have to be taken to hospital to have it removed under general anaesthetic.

What can I do to help?
Try not to allow a child under the age of three to play with toys or objects small enough to swallow or to put up her nose.

SEE ALSO:
CHOKING (p. 92), **NOSEBLEED** (p. 74)

Nosebleed

A nosebleed occurs when a small area of blood vessels on the inner surface of the nose ruptures. This can be caused by hard blowing, by sneezing, such as when your child has a common cold or hayfever, by a knock on the nose, by picking the nose, or by a foreign object in the nose; in this last instance, the blood will be accompanied by a blood-stained, foul-smelling discharge. The blood loss from a nosebleed can look very dramatic, but is usually only a small amount.

Is it serious?

A nosebleed is rarely serious. If your child has frequent nosebleeds that don't stop easily, seek medical help; if his nose bleeds after a blow to the head, dial 999/112 for emergency help.

How is it treated?

What should I do first?

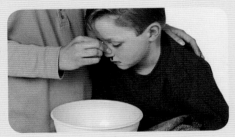

1 Don't try to staunch the blood by pushing anything into the nostrils. Sit your child down with his head forward over a basin or sink.

2 Apply firm pressure to both nostrils, gripping his nose between your thumb and forefinger just where the bone ends. Squeeze until the bleeding stops. Don't let him put his head back during a nosebleed. This allows blood to drip down the back of the nose into the stomach and can cause irritation and vomiting.

Should I seek medical help?

Seek medical advice immediately if the nosebleed fails to stop after 30 minutes and your child is dizzy. Get help urgently if there is a foreign object in your child's nose, or if the bleeds are frequent.

What might the doctor do?

✳ If your child has suffered a blow to the head, he may need to have an X-ray, to rule out the possibility of a fractured skull.

✳ If the nosebleed has failed to stop, your doctor or nurse will pack your child's nose with gauze to stem the blood flow. This will be done under a local anaesthetic. The gauze can be removed after a couple of hours.

✳ If your child has a foreign object stuck in his nose, it may be removed under local anaesthetic if necessary.

✳ If the nosebleeds are frequent, your child may be referred to an ear, nose, and throat specialist for assessment. If the recurrent nosebleeds are caused by a fragile blood vessel, the specialist may cauterize it. This involves burning off the end of the vessel, and is done under a general anaesthetic.

What can I do to help?

✳ Don't let your child blow his nose for at least three hours after a nosebleed; the bleeding might start again.

SEE ALSO:
COMMON COLD (p. 63), **HAYFEVER** (p. 89),
FOREIGN OBJECT IN NOSE (p. 73)

Styes

A stye is a pus-filled swelling on the margin of the eyelid. It is caused by an infection of one of the hair follicles from which the eyelashes grow, and it nearly always appears on the lower eyelid. It usually comes to a head and bursts within four or five days. Styes are encouraged by rubbing and pulling at the eyelashes and may also be associated with a general inflammation of the eyelids known as blepharitis. Styes are not highly infectious, but they can spread from one eye to the other.

Are they serious?

A stye can be uncomfortable and painful, but is usually harmless, and can be easily treated at home.

Possible symptoms

* Swollen, sore red area on the eyelid, which enlarges to become pus-filled

* Rubbing and pulling at eyelashes, accompanied by irritation of the eye

Common site

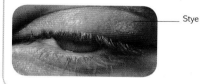

Stye

How are they treated?

What should I do first?

1 If the spot on the eyelid is merely red and sore, leave it alone and discourage your child from rubbing it. If it is painful and unsightly, keep it still with gauze held loosely in place with a bandage.

2 If the stye is pus-filled and painful, apply a ball of cotton wool squeezed out in hot water for a few minutes every two or three hours. This will soothe the pain and bring the stye to a head.

3 Once the stye has come to a head, try to release the pus and ease the pain by gently pulling out the lash at the centre of the stye with a pair of tweezers. If it won't come out, leave it, and continue with the warm compresses. As soon as the lash comes out, the pus will drain away, and the stye will get better quickly. Bathe the pus away with warm water and cotton wool.

4 Note whether the eyelids are red rimmed, with dandruff-like flakes clinging to the eyelashes. This could be an inflammation known as blepharitis. Ask your doctor if you are unsure.

Should I seek medical help?

Seek medical advice if home treatment does not improve the stye within four or five days, or if the eyelid becomes generally swollen, or if the stye is accompanied by blepharitis.

What might the doctor do?

If there is an infection of the eyelid or the eye itself, your doctor will prescribe an antibiotic ointment or eye drops. If the stye is accompanied by blepharitis, your doctor may prescribe an ointment to clear it up.

What can I do to help?

* Keep your child's facecloth and towel separate from those of the rest of the family, to avoid spreading any infection.

* Wash your hands before and after treating the stye, and discourage your child from touching the area.

Sticky eye

Sticky eye is a mild infection that is quite common during the first week of a baby's life. It is nearly always due to a foreign substance getting into the eye during delivery, possibly a drop of amniotic fluid or blood. Your baby's eye will ooze pus and when he wakes up, the eye will be gummed up.

Possible symptoms

✳ Pus coming from the inner corner of one or both of the eyes

✳ Eyelashes stuck together after sleep

Is it serious?

Sticky eye is not a serious complaint. It poses no danger to your baby's eyes, but the ailment should nevertheless always be treated promptly to prevent conjunctivitis, which is a more serious complaint of the eye membrane.

How is it treated?

What should I do first?

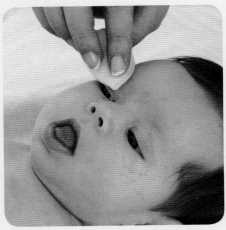

1 Wash both eyes with warm, boiled water, using a clean piece of cotton wool for each eye. Start on the inner corner of the eye and move outwards.

2 Try to stop your baby rubbing his face against the bed as he sleeps. Otherwise, the other eye may become infected from the sheet.

Should I seek medical help?
Seek medical advice immediately if your baby's eye is red. This could be conjunctivitis. Check with your doctor or nurse as soon as possible if the sticky eye does not improve within 24 hours.

What might the doctor do?
If there is an infection, your doctor will prescribe eye drops or an eye ointment, that can be applied to the eye three or four times a day.

What can I do to help?
✳ Bathe your baby's eyes frequently, whenever you notice a discharge.

✳ Change his bed sheets regularly after every sleep (particularly his pillowcases) to avoid infecting the unaffected eye.

SEE ALSO:
CONJUNCTIVITIS (p. 77)

Conjunctivitis

Conjunctivitis is an inflammation of the conjunctiva, which is the membrane covering the eyeball and the inside of the eyelid. The inflammation may be caused by a viral or bacterial infection, or by injury from a foreign object or chemicals, or it may be the result of an allergic reaction. The eyes become red and weepy, and they can be painful, very itchy, and irritated by bright light. The condition, which may affect one or both eyes, is contagious, and can also be a symptom of hayfever.

Is it serious?

Conjunctivitis is not serious, but it should always be treated by a doctor or nurse.

Possible symptoms

* Weepy, red eyes that feel sore or itchy

* Intolerance of bright light

* Discharge of pus causing eyelashes to stick together after a night's sleep

Infected eye

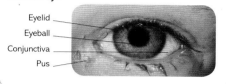

Eyelid

Eyeball

Conjunctiva

Pus

How is it treated?

What should I do first?

1 Look to see if there is a foreign object in the eye; if possible remove it.

2 Bathe each eye with cooled, previously boiled water. Using a new cotton wool ball for each eye, soak it in the water, then wipe outwards, starting from the inner corner of the eye.

3 If only one eye is affected, you can use an eye pad to prevent rubbing and further friction between the conjunctiva and other parts of the eye. Make sure that the eye pad itself does not aggravate the infection. Use a gauze pad held in place by a bandage.

4 To prevent the spread of infection, encourage your child to keep his hands clean and not to rub his eyes.

Should I seek medical help?

Seek medical advice if you suspect conjunctivitis.

What might the doctor do?

* If the condition is caused by an infection, your child may be given antibiotic eye drops

or ointment to clear it. If the infection does not respond to treatment within a few days, your child may be referred to an eye specialist.

* If the irritation is caused by an allergy, such as hayfever, your doctor will prescribe anti-inflammatory eye drops and antihistamine medication.

* If there is a foreign object in your child's eye, your doctor will remove it.

What can I do to help?

* Make your child understand that to prevent the infection from spreading, he should always keep his hands clean; he should also use a separate facecloth and towel.

* If your child suffers from hayfever, keep him away from freshly mown lawns during the worst hayfever months.

SEE ALSO:
FOREIGN OBJECT IN EYE (p. 78), **HAYFEVER** (p. 89)

Foreign object in eye

If a foreign object such as a speck of dust or grit enters your child's eye, it will water and your child will not want to open it. If you can see something moving loosely over the white part, you can try to remove it. If, however, the foreign object is embedded in the eyeball or is on the coloured part of the eye (the iris), don't touch it.

Is it serious?

Small specks of dust or grit in the eye are not serious as they are washed out naturally by the tears. But if your child's eyeball is scratched, if an object has pierced it, or if there is any kind of cut on the eyeball or eyelid, this is serious. If there is an object in the eyeball, do not try to take it out yourself. Take your child to your nearest hospital emergency department for treatment.

Possible symptoms

* ✱ Watery eye
* ✱ Reluctance to open the eye
* ✱ Pain and irritation
* ✱ A visible embedded object

How is it treated?

What should I do first?
Look closely to see whether the foreign object is moving or embedded in the eye. Encourage your child to blink a few times – this may dislodge it, as may tears if he has been crying because of the pain and irritation.

If the foreign object is embedded in the eye
Do not attempt first aid treatment yourself. Keep your child's eye closed by putting a pad over the eyelid and taping it securely in place. Go straight to the nearest hospital emergency department for treatment.

If the foreign object is not embedded in the eye
1 Ask your child to look upwards. Pull down the eyelid to see if the object is there. If it is, remove it with the corner of a clean handkerchief.

2 Expose the area beneath the top lid by holding the eyelashes and pulling them back. Remove the object with the corner of a handkerchief. If your child won't co-operate, you will need someone to help you. Seek medical assistance if necessary.

3 If these methods don't work, try to flush the foreign object out by pouring a glass of clean water across the open eye.

Should I seek medical help?
Go at once to the nearest emergency department if the eyeball is scratched, or if a foreign object has pierced the eye. Seek medical advice immediately if you cannot easily remove a floating foreign object from your child's eye.

What might the doctor do?
✱ The hospital doctor will remove the embedded foreign object from your child's eye after putting drops of a local anaesthetic into the eye.

✱ If the eyeball is scratched, the doctor will prescribe antibiotic drops to guard against infection and may bandage the eye to keep it closed for about 24 hours.

What can I do to help?
✱ After the removal of the foreign object, the pain should ease in an hour or so. If it doesn't, seek advice as soon as possible.

Teething

Teething is the term used to describe the eruption of a baby's first teeth. Teething usually begins at about the age of six or seven months, with most of the first teeth breaking through before your baby is 18 months old. Your baby will produce more saliva than usual and will dribble; he will try to cram his fingers into his mouth and chew on his fingers or any other object that he can get hold of. He may be clingy and irritable, have difficulty sleeping, and he may cry and fret more than usual. Most of these symptoms occur just before the teeth erupt. It is important to realize that the symptoms of teething do not include bronchitis, vomiting, diarrhoea, or loss of appetite. These are symptoms of an underlying illness, not teething.

Is it serious?

Teething and the symptoms associated with teething are never serious.

Possible symptoms

* Increased saliva and dribbling
* Desire to bite on any hard object
* Irritability and increased clinginess
* Swollen red area where the tooth is coming through
* Sleeplessness

Order of appearance

1   1st incisors
2   1st incisors
3   2nd incisors
4   2nd incisors
5   1st molars
6   1st molars
7   Eye teeth
8   Eye teeth
9   2nd molars
10 2nd molars

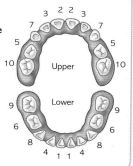

How is it treated?

What should I do first?
If you can't work out why your child is being irritable, feel his gums. If a tooth is coming through, you will feel a hard, sharp lump, and the gum area will be swollen and red.

Should I seek medical help?
You shouldn't need to consult your doctor unless your child has other symptoms that cannot be attributed to teething. Your health visitor can give you advice on how to cope with teething. Mild analgesics can be used for pain relief if necessary.

What can I do to help?
* Feed your baby often. The arrival of teeth doesn't mean a necessary speeding-up of the weaning process. Babies with teeth can still be breastfed, with no discomfort to the mother.

* Distract your child with a chilled teething ring (never freeze it or your baby may get frostbite), or a piece of carrot – something with a firm texture. Never leave your child alone with food in case he chokes.

* Try not to give your baby paracetamol. Over the course of the teething process, doses of such pain relievers could become too large. Only use pain relief on your doctor's advice.

* Rub the swollen gum with your finger. Try to avoid teething jellies that contain local anaesthetics, as they have only a temporary effect and can sometimes cause allergy.

* If your child refuses food, encourage him to eat by giving him cold, smooth foods such as yogurt, ice cream, or jelly.

Toothache

Toothache is the pain that results when a tooth is decaying. The decaying process erodes the outer protective coatings of the tooth and bores through to the nerves in the soft centre, causing pain, particularly when anything cold, hot, or sweet touches the tooth. Tooth decay and gum disease are caused by plaque, a thin film of saliva and food residue in which bacteria grow. The bacteria thrive in the presence of sugar in the mouth, which is one of the reasons why sugar in the diet is so harmful. Teeth can become resistant to the action of bacteria and sugar if they contain fluoride or if they are painted or coated with fluoride, as they would be if regularly brushed with a fluoride-containing toothpaste. This is one of the main ways to prevent tooth decay, along with good oral hygiene, and regular dental check-ups. It is important that children do not lose their first teeth through tooth decay, or a dental abscess (a complication of tooth decay in which the root of the tooth also decays). The permanent tooth may come through misaligned, if a gap is left for too long while the new tooth is developing.

Is it serious?

Toothache is not serious as long as it is treated. If untreated, an abscess may erupt, causing damage to the underlying permanent tooth, or loss of a second tooth.

How is it treated?

What should I do first?

1 If your child complains of pain in the jaw, earache, or throbbing pains in the mouth, give her paracetamol or ibuprofen to relieve the pain until you can visit the dentist.

2 Put a hot-water bottle covered in a towel against her cheek.

3 Do not apply oil of cloves or anaesthetic jellies, as they can cause damage to the gums.

Should I seek medical help?

You don't need to see a doctor, but you should consult your dentist as soon as possible for an emergency appointment.

What might the dentist do?

Your dentist will examine the tooth. It may only need to be drilled and filled, but if there is a dental abscess with pus, your dentist will drain the pus. If the tooth cannot be saved, it will be extracted, probably under a general anaesthetic, although this will depend on the age of your child.

What can I do to help?

✳ Prevent tooth decay. Use fluoride toothpastes and fluoride tablets, or drops in your child's drinks if your water is not already fluoridated.

✳ Restrict your child's sugar intake. Don't give her sweets, cakes, and biscuits, and avoid canned foods and fizzy drinks.

✳ Brush your child's teeth yourself twice a day or supervise the brushing.

✳ Once your child is three, take her for a dental check-up every six months to get her used to visits to the dentist from an early age.

✳ Encourage your child to drink lots of water after eating sweet foods, to wash most of the sugar off her teeth.

SEE ALSO:
EARACHE (p. 70), **DENTAL ABSCESS** (p. 82)

Mouth ulcers

Children suffer from a variety of mouth ulcers, all of them painful, although most are relatively harmless. Aphthous ulcers are usually small and creamy-white, and may be so painful that your child will be reluctant to eat. They are sometimes associated with stress, and may come in crops during a particularly anxious time, such as starting school.

A traumatic ulcer is larger, and usually starts as a sore patch on the inside of the cheeks, possibly after injury by biting or by the rubbing of a rough tooth. It enlarges to form a painful yellow crater. It heals very slowly and, regardless of treatment, takes 10–14 days to clear completely.

White, painful blisters on the roof of the mouth, on the gums, and inside the cheeks can be the result of a primary infection caused by the cold sore virus.

Possible symptoms

* Small, creamy-white, painful raised areas anywhere on the tongue, gums, or lining of the mouth

* Large red area with a yellow centre, particularly inside the cheeks

* White blister-like spots inside the mouth, which can sometimes be accompanied by a fever

* Loss of appetite because eating becomes too painful

Are they serious?

Mouth ulcers are not serious, but because they can be painful they sometimes cause loss of appetite and interfere with your child's eating.

How are they treated?

What should I do first?

1 If your child complains of a sore mouth or tongue, check to see if there are any areas of soreness.

2 If the ulcer is large and is inside the cheek, check for a jagged tooth that might be rubbing the cheek lining.

3 If the ulcers resemble white curds, try to wipe them off with a clean handkerchief. If this leaves red, raw patches, the ulcers could be caused by oral thrush.

4 Give your child some liquid paracetamol or ibuprofen to relieve the pain. Liquidize food to minimize chewing when ulcers are most painful.

5 If your bottlefed baby has a traumatic ulcer on the roof of her mouth, check the teat. It may be too hard for your baby's tender mouth.

Should I seek medical help?

Seek medical advice if the ulcers are very painful, or your home treatment doesn't help. See your doctor if they are recurrent. If the ulceration is caused by a jagged tooth, take your child to the dentist.

What might the doctor do?

* Your doctor will probably prescribe an anti-inflammatory cream for aphthous ulcers. The cream is not dissolved by saliva, and therefore clings to the ulcers and speeds healing.

* If your child suffers from recurrent mouth ulcers, your doctor will refer her to hospital for blood tests to see if there is an underlying cause.

SEE ALSO:
COLD SORES (p. 48)
THRUSH (p. 121)

Dental abscess

A dental abscess is a pus-filled cavity that develops at the root of a decayed tooth. In a primary tooth, an abscess can damage the underlying permanent tooth if it is left untreated. Abscesses are nearly always very painful as they are in such a confined area, and the pain does not always respond to painkillers.

Is it serious?

An abscess should be treated seriously as it causes great discomfort, and can result in a lost tooth.

Possible symptoms

* ✳ Red, inflamed lump on one side of the tooth in the gum
* ✳ Throbbing pain
* ✳ Tenderness and swelling on the affected side of the face
* ✳ Swollen neck glands
* ✳ Pain below the ear on the affected side of the face

How is it treated?

What should I do first?

1 Examine the gum around the tooth and if you notice a red lump, gently feel it with your fingertip. It will be soft and spongy because of the underlying collection of pus.

2 Give your child liquid paracetamol or ibuprofen to try to relieve the pain. Do not use local anaesthetics, such as oil of cloves. These can damage the gum margin, leading to more dental problems.

3 Rinse your child's mouth with water to speed the bursting of the abscess, and to wash away any pus that has seeped out.

4 Apply a covered hot-water bottle to your child's cheek to soothe the pain.

Should I seek medical help?
Consult your dentist as soon as possible.

What might the dentist do?
✳ The dentist will drain the pus by either opening the gum or removing the tooth if there is no possibility of saving it. Both will be done under local anaesthetic.

✳ Your dentist will prescribe a course of antibiotics to eradicate the infection. Your child may also be prescribed a mouthwash to use three or four times a day until the wound has healed.

What can I do to help?
✳ Maintain regular toothbrushing to minimize tooth decay.

✳ Take your child to the dentist regularly from the age of three.

✳ Cut down on sweets, sugary foods, and fizzy drinks in your child's diet.

SEE ALSO:
EARACHE (p. 70)
TOOTHACHE (p. 80)

Chapter 5

Respiratory system

Diseases of the respiratory system
can range from the common and minor,
such as coughs, to the more serious, such
as asthma. All need careful handling, as
described in the entries that follow.

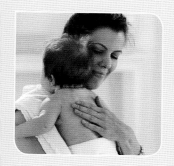

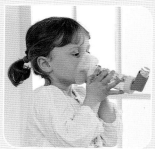

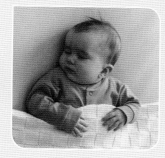

Diagnosis guide

Because respiratory ailments vary widely from minor to serious, it is particularly important to be able to spot and treat them quickly. To use this section, look for the symptom most similar to the one your child is suffering from then turn to the relevant entry. See also p. 13 for a list of symptoms requiring emergency treatment.

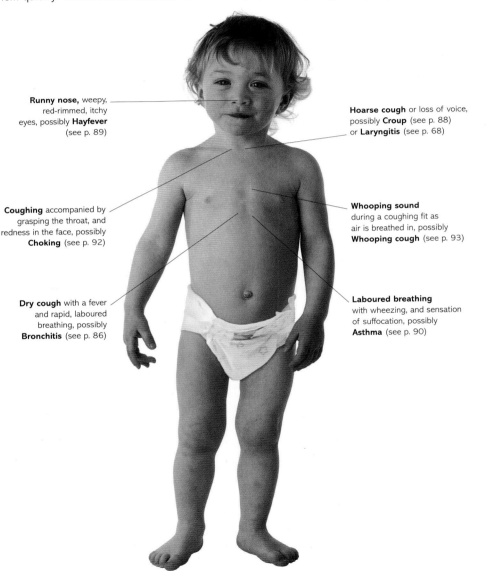

Runny nose, weepy, red-rimmed, itchy eyes, possibly **Hayfever** (see p. 89)

Hoarse cough or loss of voice, possibly **Croup** (see p. 88) or **Laryngitis** (see p. 68)

Coughing accompanied by grasping the throat, and redness in the face, possibly **Choking** (see p. 92)

Whooping sound during a coughing fit as air is breathed in, possibly **Whooping cough** (see p. 93)

Dry cough with a fever and rapid, laboured breathing, possibly **Bronchitis** (see p. 86)

Laboured breathing with wheezing, and sensation of suffocation, possibly **Asthma** (see p. 90)

Cough

A cough is either a symptom of a disease, or the body's way of reacting to an irritant in the throat or air passages. A wet cough or productive cough may bring up phlegm from the chest and clear mucus from the air passages, for example, during an attack of asthma or whooping cough. A dry cough, which produces no phlegm, does not always have an obvious cause. The irritation provoking the cough may be mucus from chronically infected sinuses or nasal discharge from a common cold, or it may also be the body's way of bringing up a foreign object stuck in the windpipe. If your child is exposed to cigarette smoke, the smoke may irritate his throat and cause a cough. Children can also sometimes adopt a cough as an attention-seeking device.

Is it serious?

A cough is not usually serious, although it can be irritating. However, a cough that causes breathing difficulties is serious and should be treated as an emergency.

How is it treated?

What should I do first?

1 If your child is coughing up phlegm, lay him over your lap on his stomach. Pat him gently on the back to help him bring up the phlegm.

2 If you think that your child has a foreign object in his throat, see Choking (p. 92).

3 If he is coughing at night, prop him up with pillows. This will stop mucus or nasal discharge from dribbling down the throat. To soothe his throat, give hot lemon sweetened with honey.

Should I seek medical help?

Seek medical advice if the cough doesn't get better after three or four days, or if your child is not getting any sleep. If you cannot remove a foreign object from his throat or he has difficulty breathing, dial 999/112 for emergency help.

What might the doctor do?

* If your child's cough is part of an infection such as tonsillitis or croup, your doctor may prescribe antibiotics.

* Your doctor may prescribe nose drops to administer sparingly to your child before he goes to bed. These drops ease congestion and prevent mucus from dribbling down the back of his throat.

* If your child is suffering from a viral infection, your doctor or nurse will advise you on how to relieve symptoms.

* If the cough is part of an asthmatic condition, your doctor may prescribe bronchodilator drugs.

* Your doctor may also advise you about cough medicines for your child.

What can I do to help?

* Keep your child warm to help prevent any minor infection from spreading into the lungs, but don't overheat the room.

* Keep the air in his room moist by leaving a window open.

* Avoid giving him cough suppressants.

SEE ALSO:

ASTHMA (p. 90)

BRONCHITIS (p. 86)

CHOKING (p. 92)

COMMON COLD (p. 63)

CROUP (p. 88)

TONSILLITIS (p. 67)

WHOOPING COUGH (p. 93)

Bronchitis

Bronchitis is inflammation of the membranes
that line the airways leading to the lungs.
It arises when a minor infection, such as a
common cold, reduces resistance to infection.
The lining of the airways swells and mucus
builds up, making breathing difficult. A hacking
cough produces phlegm which, if the child
swallows it, may make him vomit.

Is it serious?

Most children recover fully within a week.
In those over a year old, bronchitis is not
usually serious, but in rare cases it may
require hospitalization.

Possible symptoms

* ✳ Fever
* ✳ Dry, hacking cough, changing to a cough
  that produces green or yellow phlegm
* ✳ Rapid breathing, over 40 breaths
  per minute, with wheezing
* ✳ Breathing difficulties
* ✳ Loss of appetite
* ✳ Vomiting with the cough
* ✳ Blueness of the lips and tongue

How is it treated?

What should I do first?
1 If your child has recently had a cold, sore
throat, sinusitis, or an ear infection, and his
condition worsens, take his temperature. If he
has a fever, take his temperature every three
to four hours, and try to bring it down by giving
him paracetamol or ibuprofen.

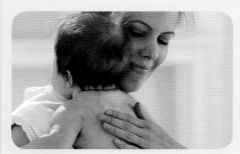

2 If he is coughing, check for phlegm. If there is,
encourage him to cough it up. If he can't do this,
pat him on the back during the coughing attack.

3 Give your child liquids, to prevent dehydration.
Avoid patent cough suppressants if there is
phlegm, as it needs to be coughed up.

Should I seek medical help?
Dial 999/112 for emergency help if he has
difficulty breathing, is drawing in his chest with
every breath, or if there is any sign of blueness
around his lips and on his tongue. Always seek
medical advice if his infection gets worse.

What might the doctor do?
* ✳ If your child is in great distress because of
breathing difficulties, he will be admitted to
hospital, so that he can be given either oxygen
to help with breathing, or intravenous fluids to
prevent dehydration.

* ✳ Your doctor will prescribe antibiotics if a
bacterial infection is present. If your child's
bronchitis is caused by a virus, you will be
advised on nursing procedures because there
is no specific medication.

SEE ALSO:
COMMON COLD (p. 63), **COUGH** (p. 85), **SINUSITIS** (p. 65),
SORE THROAT (p. 66), **VOMITING** (p. 100)

Influenza

Influenza (flu), like the common cold, is caused by a virus and has no known cure. It lasts around five to seven days. Unless there is a secondary infection, treatment of the symptoms is usually all that is necessary in most cases.

Is it serious?

It is rare for serious complications to occur with influenza. However, natural resistance is reduced and a secondary infection, such as pneumonia, earache, bronchitis, or sinusitis, could result. Influenza is always serious in a child who has asthma, or a condition such as diabetes mellitus.

Possible symptoms

* Runny nose
* Sore throat
* Cough
* Fever
* Shivering
* Aches and pains
* Diarrhoea, vomiting, or nausea
* Weakness and lethargy

How is it treated?

What should I do first?

1 Check your child's temperature every three to four hours. If it has not come down after 36 hours, seek medical advice.

2 Give your child paracetamol or ibuprofen, and put him to bed.

3 Don't force your child to eat, but make sure he gets plenty to drink.

Should I seek medical help?

Seek medical advice immediately if your child's temperature fails to come down within 36 hours, or if you notice a deterioration in his condition. Watch out for a worsening cough, which may suggest a chest infection, or yellow pus discharge from the nose, which may indicate sinusitis or earache.

What might the doctor do?

If there is a secondary infection, your child may need antibiotics.

What can I do to help?

* Your child should rest in bed in a warm room. As soon as he feels better, let him get up, but make him rest if his temperature rises again.

* Use paper tissues and dispose of them after each use.

* You might consider protecting your child with an annual influenza vaccine.

* If, after your child should have recovered, his temperature rises and he vomits, seek medical advice immediately. A rare but serious illness, Reye's syndrome, could be the cause.

SEE ALSO:

ASTHMA (p. 90)
BRONCHITIS (p. 86)
COMMON COLD (p. 63)
COUGH (p. 85)
EARACHE (p. 70)
FEVER (p. 26)

Croup

Croup is the name given to the sound made when air is breathed in through a constricted windpipe, past inflamed vocal cords. It usually occurs only in young children up to the age of about four, who are susceptible because their air passages (bronchi) are narrow, and become blocked with mucus when they are inflamed – most commonly because of a virus such as a common cold, or an infection such as bronchitis. In older children, the condition is less serious, and is known as laryngitis. The first attack of croup can come quickly, usually at night, and it may last for a couple of hours. Your child will have a croaking, barking cough, and laboured breathing.

Possible symptoms

* ✳ Croaking cough
* ✳ Laboured breathing when the lower chest caves in at every inhalation
* ✳ Wheezing
* ✳ Face colour becoming grey or blue

Is it serious?

If your child has a severe attack of croup, she could develop breathing difficulties. This should be treated as an emergency.

How is it treated?

What should I do first?
1 Stay calm and soothe your child so that she won't panic and make her breathing more difficult.

2 Your child's air passages will be soothed by moist air. If the air outside is cool and damp, take her to the window, and get her to take a deep breath of air, or take her into the bathroom, and turn on the hot taps to build up a steamy atmosphere.

3 Prop your child up comfortably in bed with pillows or hold her on your lap. It will be easier for her to breathe if she is sitting up.

Should I seek medical help?
Dial 999/112 for emergency help if your child's skin turns grey or blue and she has to fight for breath. Seek medical help as soon as possible if your child has an attack of croup.

What might the doctor do?
✳ If necessary, your doctor will prescribe antibiotics to eradicate any underlying infection.

✳ Your doctor will give you advice on what to do should your child have another attack.

What can I do to help?
If any further attacks occur, stay with your child, and follow the instructions your doctor has given you.

SEE ALSO:
BRONCHITIS (p. 86)
COMMON COLD (p. 63)
LARYNGITIS (p. 68)

Hayfever

Hayfever is an allergic reaction that occurs in the mucus membranes of the nose and eyelids. The condition is also known as allergic rhinitis, and causes sneezing, a runny nose, and itchy, watery eyes. It occurs in spring and summer, and is usually due to a reaction to pollens from flowers, grasses, and trees. Children who suffer from hayfever can become mouth-breathers because their nose is mostly blocked. Hayfever does not tend to occur before the age of five, but it can start or stop at any time, and can run in families. Some children who are allergic to animals and house dust, as well as pollens, suffer all year round from hayfever; this condition is called perennial allergic rhinitis.

Possible symptoms

* Sneezing
* Runny nose with clear discharge
* Itchy, watery, red-rimmed eyes

Is it serious?

It is difficult for most hayfever sufferers to avoid symptoms, as they are sensitive to more than one pollen. Although it can be troublesome, hayfever does not have any serious or life-threatening consequences.

How is it treated?

What should I do first?

1 If your child is sneezing a lot, check her temperature to make sure she isn't ill with an infection such as influenza or a common cold.

2 Discourage your child from rubbing her eyes; this will make them worse. To ease irritation, bathe her eyes with cooled, previously boiled water.

Should I seek medical help?

Seek medical advice as soon as possible if you think your child may be suffering from a more serious infection, or if the hayfever is making her miserable.

What might the doctor do?

* Decongestant nasal drops or antihistamine spray, liquid, or tablets will probably be prescribed to relieve your child's symptoms.

* If your child's condition is severe, she may need to have a series of skin tests to track down the allergen that is causing the symptoms. Once the allergens have been identified, a special vaccine can be made for her, and a course of desensitizing injections can be given over a period of weeks to protect her. However, these vaccines don't always work, and have to be given during the winter.

What can I do to help?

* Watch the pollen count each day, and if it is high discourage your child from playing near freshly mown grassland.

* Avoid feathers in your child's bedding and fluff in her clothing.

* Keep your house as dust-free as possible. Even if your child isn't allergic to dust, a dusty atmosphere makes the condition worse.

* Prepare an emergency pack for outings. It should contain paper handkerchiefs, eye drops, a moist towel to soothe your child's eyes, and whatever medication has been prescribed.

SEE ALSO:

ASTHMA (p. 90), **COMMON COLD** (p. 63), **INFLUENZA** (p. 87)

Asthma

Asthma is an allergic disease that affects the air passages (bronchi). When the allergic reaction takes place, the bronchi constrict and become clogged with mucus, making breathing difficult. An asthma attack can be very frightening for a young child because the feeling of suffocation can cause panic, making breathing even more difficult. The initial cause of the allergic reaction, the allergen, is usually airborne – pollen or house dust, for example. Emotional stress and exercise can also bring on an attack.

Asthma tends to run in families, and can be accompanied by other allergic diseases, such as eczema. However, more than half of the children who suffer from asthma eventually grow out of it by early adulthood; in many of the rest, the attacks become less severe as they grow older.

Many babies under one year wheeze if they suffer from bronchiolitis, when their small air passages become inflamed. These babies are not necessarily suffering from asthma; as they grow and their air passages widen, the wheezing will stop. Infection, rather than an allergic reaction, is the usual cause of this.

Possible symptoms

✳ Laboured breathing: when breathing out becomes difficult, and the abdomen may be drawn inward with the effort of breathing in

✳ Sensation of suffocation

✳ Wheezing

✳ Persistent cough

✳ Blueness around the lips (cyanosis) due to lack of oxygen

Affected area

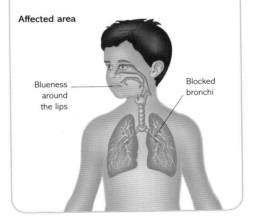

Blueness around the lips

Blocked bronchi

Is it serious?

Asthma attacks can be frightening, but with medication and advice from your doctor, your child should suffer no serious complications.

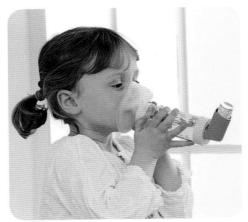

Spacer Using a spacer device with the inhaler makes it easier for younger children to inhale the drug, which is usually delivered as a spray. The spacer holds the drug before it is inhaled.

How is it treated?

What should I do first?

1 Dial 999/112 for emergency help if your child is having her first asthma attack.

2 If your child is diagnosed as having asthma and bronchodilator medicine has been prescribed, help her to use it as instructed.

3 If the attack occurs when your child is in bed, sit her up, propped up with pillows; otherwise, make her sit on a chair with her arms braced against the back to take the weight off her chest; allowing the chest muscles to force air out.

4 Stay calm; a show of anxiety from you will only make her more upset.

5 Seek medical help if your child doesn't respond to the bronchodilator medicine.

Should I seek medical help?

Dial 999/112 for emergency help if your child is having her first asthma attack. If any further attacks occur, stay with your child and follow the instructions you have been given.

What might the doctor do?

* Your child will probably be treated with a bronchodilator drug, which is inhaled directly into the bronchi and gets right to the site of the restriction. A severe attack may require treatment in hospital, where larger doses of bronchodilator drugs may be given. Your child will also be given a spacer device to use with the inhaler. This makes the inhaler easier to cope with, especially for young children.

* If there is some evidence of a chest infection, antibiotics will be prescribed.

* Your doctor will measure your child's peak expiry flow rate (PEFR) to monitor her condition.

* Your doctor will discuss prevention of further attacks and may try to determine the allergen. You will be given a supply of a bronchodilator drug in an inhaler with a spacer. This should be given as soon as an attack begins. You will

be asked to tell your doctor if your child has a severe attack, or if an attack does not respond to two doses of the bronchodilator.

* Your doctor may prescribe a steroid drug if other simpler measures don't prevent further attacks. A small dose of steroid may be inhaled three or four times a day or, if this is not effective, a larger dose will be given in tablet form.

* Your health visitor can help you monitor the severity and frequency of your child's attacks, and give general advice about ongoing treatment.

What can I do to help?

* Help your doctor if he fails to pinpoint the allergen. Notice when the attacks occur and at what time of the day or year. Avoid obvious allergens, such as feather pillows, and keep the dust down in your house by vacuuming floors and damp-dusting surfaces often.

* Many asthmatics are allergic to animals. If you have a pet, ask a friend to look after it for a while and see if your child's attacks are reduced.

* Make sure your child has the prescribed drugs nearby at all times. Inform her school about her asthma.

* Ask to be referred to a physiotherapist so that your child can learn breathing exercises to help her remain calm during an attack.

* Encourage your child to stand and sit up straight so that her lungs have more space. Don't allow her to become overweight as this will put an extra burden on her lungs.

* Moderate exercise can help her breathing, but too much can bring on an asthma attack. Swimming, however, can be especially helpful.

* Do not smoke, or allow smoking in your home or anywhere near your child.

SEE ALSO:
ECZEMA (p. 51), **HAYFEVER** (p. 89)

Choking

Choking is the blockage of the airway by a foreign object that has entered the airway instead of the passage to the stomach. If there is enough air getting through to the lungs, your child should be able to cough it back up into the mouth.

Is it serious?

If your child is coughing and gasping for breath, or turning red then blue in the face, treat it as an emergency and dial 999/112 for emergency help. If the airway is totally blocked, he will lose consciousness and stop breathing; if this happens, dial 999/112 for emergency help and start CPR (rescue breathing and chest compressions).

Possible symptoms

✳ Coughing

✳ Grasping the throat

✳ Redness, followed by blueness in the face – the blood vessels in the neck and face may stand out

How is it treated?

If your baby is choking

1 Lay him along your forearm, with his head lower than his chest and his chin supported between your fingers. Give up to five sharp blows on the middle of his back with your other hand.

2 If the object appears in his mouth, pick it out. Hold your baby steady with your other hand to prevent him from re-inhaling the object.

3 If the object doesn't come out give him alternate back slaps and chest thrusts. To do chest thrusts, put two fingers on his lower breastbone, just below the nipple line, and thrust downwards. Check his mouth to see if the obstruction has cleared.

4 Repeat three times, and if the object does not come out dial 999/112 for emergency help.

If your child is choking

1 Bend him forward with his head lower than his chest. Give him up to five firm blows between his shoulders.

2 If the foreign object appears in your child's mouth, ask him to spit it out.

3 If the object doesn't come out, give your child alternating back blows and abdominal thrusts. To do abdominal thrusts, stand behind him and make a fist with one hand. Curve it around his front and place it against his central upper abdomen. Grasp your fist with your other hand, then press both together into his abdomen in a quick upward thrusting movement. Check his mouth to see if the obstruction has cleared.

4 Repeat three times, and if the object does not come out dial 999/112 for emergency help.

Should I seek medical help?

If the obstruction has not cleared, and your baby or child turns blue or loses consciousness, dial 999/112 for emergency help immediately and inform ambulance control of his condition. If he is conscious, continue giving your baby alternate back blows and chest thrusts, or your child back blows and abdominal thrusts, while waiting for emergency help. If your baby or child loses consciousness or stops breathing, get emergency advice by telephone about what you can do until help arrives. Start CPR and continue until help arrives.

Whooping cough

Whooping cough is one of the most dangerous childhood diseases, especially in babies under a year old.

It begins as an ordinary cold with a cough. The coughing becomes severe, with spasmodic bouts that make it difficult to breathe. When your child manages to draw breath, there is a whooping sound as air is drawn in past the swollen larynx. Breathing difficulties are even greater for babies, who may never develop the technique of whooping to get air into their lungs. Sometimes vomiting occurs after a coughing bout. The coughing phase of whooping cough can last for up to 10 weeks. The risk of developing a secondary infection, such as bronchitis, is high after this disease.

Possible symptoms

* Common cold-like symptoms of runny nose, fever, and aches and pains
* Excessive coughing, with a characteristic "whoop" as the child struggles to draw breath
* Vomiting after a coughing bout
* Sleeplessness because of coughing

Is it serious?

It is serious, especially in babies. Vomiting can cause dehydration. A severe attack can damage the lungs and cause recurrent bronchial infections.

How is it treated?

What should I do first?

1 If your child's cold fails to improve and his cough worsens, put him to bed and seek medical help.

2 If you suspect your baby has whooping cough, consult your doctor immediately. If you suspect your child has it, keep him from school until you have seen your doctor.

3 If he is having a long coughing bout, sit him up and hold him so that he is leaning slightly forward. Hold a bowl so that he can spit any phlegm into it. Warm, moist inhalations help.

Should I seek medical help?

Seek medical help immediately if you suspect whooping cough.

What might the doctor do?

* Your doctor may prescribe antibiotics to limit your child's infectiousness. He may need to take a throat swab from your baby to diagnose whooping cough because babies rarely whoop.

* Your doctor will keep a close check on a baby with whooping cough and if it is severe, may recommend hospitalization.

* Your doctor will make sure you know how to hold your child during a coughing attack. You may be advised to raise the foot of your baby's cot.

What can I do to help?

* Put bowls everywhere so that your child can spit up phlegm or vomit. If he vomits after coughing, give him small meals and drinks to help him keep some nourishment down.

* Sleep in the room with him so that he is never alone during a coughing bout.

* If, afterwards, he seems sick and is breathing with difficulty, seek medical advice immediately.

* Don't give cough medication without advice.

SEE ALSO:
BRONCHITIS (p. 86)
VOMITING (p. 100)

Cot death

Sudden infant death syndrome (SIDS), or cot death, is the sudden and often unexplained death of a seemingly healthy baby. There is no single known cause of cot death, although research has shown that some deaths can be the result of an abnormality in the breathing and heart rate. The current areas of research include the development of a baby's temperature control mechanism and respiratory system in the first six months, and the recent discovery that an inherited enzyme deficiency may be responsible for around one per cent of cases. Studies connecting SIDS with flame-retardant chemicals in cot mattresses have, so far, proven inconclusive.

The death of an infant from SIDS is a particularly distressing experience. Severe grief can be compounded by intense feelings of guilt and misplaced blame, and affect family relationships. Parents of cot death infants may have to discuss the incident with the police and be prepared for post-mortem examination of the baby. Your doctor, paediatrician, and health visitor should all provide valuable support and counselling in this situation, and talking to other parents who have also experienced a cot death, or to a professional organization, can help, too.

Possible symptoms

* Common cold-like symptom of stuffy nose
* Inexplicable weight loss

How can it be prevented?

What should I do?
While the causes of cot death are not clear, there are ways in which you can reduce the risks.

* Always put your baby to sleep on her back, never on her front. Babies who sleep on their backs are at reduced risk of cot death. This will also help control your baby's body temperature.

* Don't wrap her in too many nightclothes or bedclothes, especially during winter, or put her to bed in a room that is too warm. Use a thermostatically controlled heater in her room so that temperatures do not rise too high, or drop too low. Make sure she has enough blankets – a sheet and two blankets is sufficient in a room temperature of 16°C (61°F). Use fewer bedclothes if the temperature is higher – no more than one sheet and no blanket on a warm night of 24°C (75°F).

* Do not smoke during pregnancy and after your child is born – fathers, too.

* Ban smokers from the house.

* Be careful not to swaddle or tuck your baby in. Don't use baby nests, sheepskins, duvets, and cot bumpers as they all prevent heat loss.

* Whenever possible, breastfeed rather than bottlefeed your baby.

* Avoid taking unnecessary drugs during pregnancy.

* If you think your baby is unwell, contact your doctor. If she has a fever, don't increase the wrapping – reduce it so she can lose heat. After a minor illness, keep a closer eye than usual on her for several days until the symptoms disappear.

FOR HELP AND ADVICE CONTACT:
Foundation for the Study of Infant Death (FSID)
11 Belgrave Road, London SW1V 1RB
020 7802 3200
www.fsid.org.uk

Chapter 6

Digestion

The digestive system is responsible for **processing food** and includes various organs, such as the salivary glands, liver, and pancreas. The **ailments** that can affect digestion include **colic, food poisoning,** and **gastroenteritis.** All are described in detail, with useful practical suggestions.

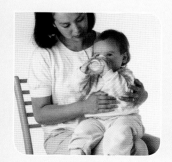

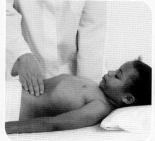

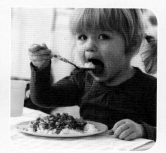

Diagnosis guide

Because young children are prone to a variety of acute digestive complaints, it is important that you are able to deal with them before your child's condition deteriorates. To use this section, look for the symptom most similar to the one that your child is suffering from, then turn to the relevant entry. See also p. 13 for a list of symptoms requiring emergency treatment.

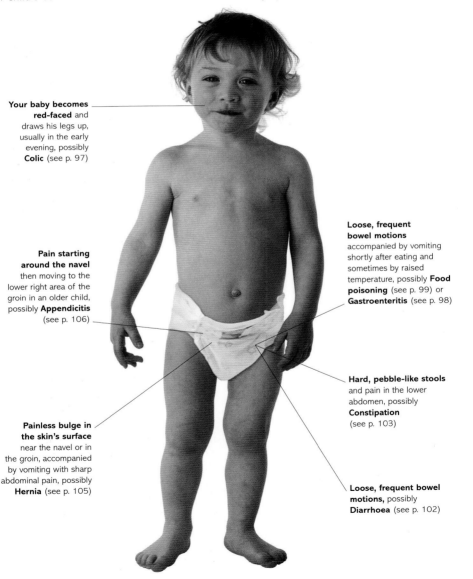

Your baby becomes red-faced and draws his legs up, usually in the early evening, possibly **Colic** (see p. 97)

Pain starting around the navel then moving to the lower right area of the groin in an older child, possibly **Appendicitis** (see p. 106)

Painless bulge in the skin's surface near the navel or in the groin, accompanied by vomiting with sharp abdominal pain, possibly **Hernia** (see p. 105)

Loose, frequent bowel motions accompanied by vomiting shortly after eating and sometimes by raised temperature, possibly **Food poisoning** (see p. 99) or **Gastroenteritis** (see p. 98)

Hard, pebble-like stools and pain in the lower abdomen, possibly **Constipation** (see p. 103)

Loose, frequent bowel motions, possibly **Diarrhoea** (see p. 102)

Colic

Colic, as applied to a baby under four months of age, describes a crying spell during which the baby's face becomes very red, and both legs are drawn up to her stomach as if she is in great pain. These crying spells usually happen during the early evenings; the baby is generally contented during the rest of the day. The crying can reach screaming pitch and may last from one to three hours. Remember your baby will not respond to soothing techniques that usually work at other times. Colic is so common that it is regarded by paediatricians as normal, but for parents it can be difficult to endure. The cause of the apparent spasmodic pain is not known. It is often at its worst at three months of age but disappears by four months.

Possible symptoms

* Your baby cannot settle in the early evening and cries no matter what you do to calm her

* She becomes red-faced and draws her legs up into her stomach as if in pain

* She may wake from a short sleep with a startled cry

Is it serious?

The fact that your baby is contented during the rest of the day means that this crying bout is not related to a serious physical problem.

How is it treated?

What should I do first?

1 Try all the methods of soothing your baby that you know work at other times of the day. This may mean you are constantly offering the breast or bottle, changing nappies, winding, nursing, and rocking your baby. You might even be walking with the baby held over the shoulder, putting her in a sling against your body, playing music to give a constant background noise, or walking her in a pram.

2 Try using a dummy – your baby may need to suck all the time.

3 Don't use any patent medicines without your doctor's advice.

4 Bathe your baby at this difficult time of the day. A warm bath relaxes most babies.

Should I seek medical help?

Seek medical advice if you find you cannot cope with the nightly crying sessions.

What might the doctor do?

* Your doctor or nurse can reassure you that your baby is healthy, and that she will grow out of the colic eventually.

* Health visitors can provide valuable advice and counselling while your baby is still having attacks.

What can I do to help?

* Make sure you look after yourself. You will be able to cope better if you get as much sleep as you possibly can during the day while your baby sleeps.

* Invite good friends in to share that time of the evening with you; a relaxed atmosphere may calm both you and your baby.

* Talk to other parents who have had colicky babies. Once you realize that colic attacks do pass, you may find them easier to bear.

Gastroenteritis

Gastroenteritis is inflammation of the stomach and intestines caused in children mostly by the rotavirus, which can be inhaled and spreads easily. It may also be caused by direct infection of the intestines, usually from contaminated food (food poisoning) or a parasite (sometimes known as dysentery). In some cases, it may be an indication of influenza. Among babies, it is most common in bottlefed babies, and is usually the result of poor sterilization of feeding equipment.

Possible symptoms

✳ Vomiting

✳ Nausea

✳ Diarrhoea

✳ Abdominal cramps

✳ Loss of appetite

✳ Fever

Is it serious?

Most attacks are mild, but severe gastroenteritis is very serious in children, especially babies, because vomiting and diarrhoea can rapidly lead to dehydration.

How is it treated?

What should I do first?

1 Stop all foods and milk and give your child only water in small amounts every 15 minutes.

2 Put your child to bed with a bowl by the bed in case he vomits.

3 Make sure he washes his hands after going to the toilet.

Should I seek medical help?

Seek medical advice immediately if your child has diarrhoea and vomiting for more than six hours, and you cannot bring them under control with a fluids-only diet.

What might the doctor do?

✳ Your doctor or nurse will probably prescribe a special powder containing glucose and essential minerals to be added to your child's drinks, to replace what has been lost through vomiting and diarrhoea. To avoid dehydration, your child should be given 200ml (7fl oz) of water for every kilogram (2lb) of his body weight in the first 24 hours of diarrhoea and vomiting.

✳ Your doctor or nurse will recommend bed-rest and a liquid diet until the vomiting and diarrhoea have subsided.

✳ For a bottlefed baby, your doctor or nurse may suggest that you replace milk feeds with a glucose solution, and give you a regime for reintroducing formula feeds.

✳ If your baby is seriously ill, your doctor may admit him to hospital.

What can I do to help?

✳ Be meticulous about hygiene.

✳ Avoid giving your child acidic drinks, such as orange juice. They may irritate the stomach further.

✳ Reintroduce foods slowly when your child seems interested, starting with easily digested foods, such as jellies, yogurt, soups, and non-fatty foods.

✳ If he refuses to drink enough fluids, or doesn't like glucose powder, give him cubes of melon.

SEE ALSO:

DIARRHOEA (p. 102), **FOOD POISONING** (p. 99), **INFLUENZA** (p. 87), **VOMITING** (p. 100)

Food poisoning

This is a form of gastroenteritis caused by eating food contaminated with poisons, usually from bacteria. *E. coli* is the bacterium most commonly responsible for food poisoning among babies; salmonella and *staphylococcii* are also fairly common. Symptoms can also arise from eating chemicals, insecticides, or even certain plants.

Is it serious?

In a baby, it is serious because it can rapidly lead to dehydration.

Possible symptoms

* Abdominal cramps
* Fever or vomiting
* Frequent, loose stools that may contain blood, pus, or mucus
* Muscular weakness and chills

How is it treated?

What should I do first?

1 If your child is vomiting and has diarrhoea, measure his temperature to see if he has a fever. Check his stools for mucus or blood.

2 Put him to bed and stop all foods, but keep offering him frequent small drinks of water.

3 Try to determine the cause of the symptoms.

Should I seek medical help?

Seek medical advice immediately if vomiting and diarrhoea continue for more than six hours and you cannot bring them under control with a fluids-only diet. Consult your doctor immediately if your child's condition has not improved within 24 hours. If you suspect that he has drunk an insecticide or eaten a poisonous plant dial 999/112 for emergency help. Keep the suspected poison.

What might the doctor do?

* In the majority of cases there is no special treatment for food poisoning except to replace fluids and salts lost through diarrhoea and vomiting. Your doctor or nurse will probably prescribe a powder containing glucose and essential minerals to be added to your child's drinks, and to replace all milk feeds in a bottlefed baby.

* If your child is in danger of dehydration, your doctor will admit him to hospital. If vomiting is severe, he may give him an injection of an antiemetic (antivomiting) drug.

What can I do to help?

* Place a bowl next to your child's bed for him to vomit into, so that he doesn't have to run to the toilet.

* Keep him cool with a covered icepack or a damp face cloth if he has a fever.

* Help your child rinse his mouth out with water after he has vomited.

* Reintroduce foods that are easily digested, such as soups, yogurt, and jellies.

* Be meticulous about hygiene.

* To prevent food poisoning, defrost foods well before cooking, refrigerate all cooked food, and reheat it thoroughly.

SEE ALSO:

DIARRHOEA (p. 102)

FEVER (p. 26)

GASTROENTERITIS (p. 98)

VOMITING (p. 100)

Vomiting

Consult your doctor immediately if your child continues to vomit over a six-hour period; if the vomiting is accompanied by diarrhoea or a fever; or if the vomiting is accompanied by any other symptoms, such as earache.

Vomiting is the violent expulsion of the contents of the stomach through the mouth. A baby may posset up small quantities of curdled milk after a feed – this is normal and harmless

and should not be confused with vomiting. Vomiting has many causes (see below), but in the majority of cases there is little warning, and after a single bout your child should be comfortable and back to normal again. Vomiting can be a symptom of a specific disorder of the stomach, such as pyloric stenosis, or a symptom of an infection, such as an ear infection. It frequently accompanies a fever, and even the common cold can cause vomiting

Symptoms and causes

ACCOMPANYING SYMPTOMS	COMMON CAUSES
Your baby often brings up a little milk during or after a feed, but seems contented, feeds well, and is gaining weight.	This regurgitation of a little milk – possetting – is normal and harmless.
Your baby is hungry and seems well, but vomits during, or immediately after, his feed.	Solids given before he can chew properly may be the cause. Until your baby is about eight months old, give puréed foods.
Your baby has a runny or blocked nose, snuffly breathing, or a cough.	A Common cold (p. 63) can make your baby vomit if he swallows a lot of mucus. A Cough (p. 85) may also make him vomit.
Your bottlefed or weaned baby, or child, seems unwell and has passed frequent, watery stools.	**Consult your doctor immediately.** Your baby may have Gastroenteritis (p. 98). An older child may have Food poisoning (p. 99).
Your child seems unwell, looks flushed, and feels hot.	An infection is the most likely cause. See Fever (p. 26).
When travelling, your child seems pale and quiet, and complains of nausea.	Travel sickness is the most likely cause.
Your child complains of a severe headache on one side of his forehead.	He could have Migraine (p. 117).
Your child has abdominal pain around the navel, and to the lower right side of his groin.	**Consult your doctor immediately.** Your child could have Appendicitis (p. 106).
Your baby is in severe pain and is passing stools that contain blood and mucus resembling redcurrant jelly.	**Consult your doctor immediately.** Your baby could have a bowel blockage known as intussusception.
Your child cannot bend his neck forward without pain, and turns away from bright light.	**Consult your doctor immediately.** Your child may have Meningitis (p. 118).

if your child swallows enough nasal discharge to irritate his stomach. If your child has a bad cough, this can also sometimes cause him to vomit up food that he has recently eaten. Other possible causes of vomiting include appendicitis, meningitis, migraine, headaches, food poisoning, and travel sickness. Children can also occasionally vomit due to excitement and anticipation, although this is generally limited to toddlers.

Is it serious?

Vomiting should always be taken seriously because it can rapidly cause dehydration, particularly in a baby or young child.

How is it treated?

What should I do first?

1 Put your child to bed, and place a bowl for him to vomit into within easy reach.

2 Give your child frequent, small amounts of water to prevent dehydration, every 10–15 minutes.

3 Check your child's temperature to see if he also has a fever. Keep him cool by wiping his face with a cool, damp cloth.

4 Have him brush his teeth to take away the taste.

Should I seek medical help?

Seek medical advice if your child continues to vomit over a six-hour period. Get help immediately if the vomiting is accompanied by diarrhoea or a fever over 38°C (100.4°F), or if the vomiting is accompanied by any other worrying symptoms.

What might the doctor do?

* Your doctor will diagnose the cause of the vomiting, and treat your child accordingly, making sure there is no danger of dehydration.

* Your child may be admitted to hospital to be given fluids intravenously if he is in danger of becoming dehydrated.

What can I do to help?

* Give your child plenty of his favourite drinks, but avoid orange juice and other acidic juices, and don't give him milk.

* Feed your child bland foods when the nausea and vomiting have passed. Reintroduce solid foods slowly.

SEE ALSO :
APPENDICITIS (p. 106)
COMMON COLD (p. 63)
DIARRHOEA (p. 102)
EARACHE (p. 70)
FEVER (p. 26)
FOOD POISONING (p. 99)
HEADACHE (p. 116)
MENINGITIS (p. 118)
MIGRAINE (p. 117)

Diarrhoea

Diarrhoea is the frequent passage of loose, watery stools, and is a sign of irritation of the intestines. Once babies begin to take solid foods, bowel motions become firmer and more regular. Loose, frequent stools can result when a baby or child eats too much of a food that is rich in dietary fibre, such as fruit, or they may be a symptom of an infection. Food may have been contaminated with bacteria (food poisoning), or an infection from contaminated stools may have been spread to the mouth by unwashed hands. Diarrhoea can also be the symptom of a non-intestinal infection, such as influenza, when it may be accompanied by fever.

Ironically, stools similar to those of diarrhoea may be caused by constipation. If an older child soils herself with liquid stools, this may be because of a type of constipation known as encopresis.

Is it serious?

Diarrhoea in a baby is always serious because of the dangers of dehydration. Diarrhoea accompanied by vomiting in a young child is also serious for the same reason, especially if accompanied by fever and sweating. Diarrhoea in which the stools are greasy and foul-smelling can be a symptom of cystic fibrosis.

How is it treated?

What should I do first?

1 If your baby is under one year old and has had diarrhoea for six hours, consult your doctor as soon as possible.

2 Don't give an older child any food or milk, but give frequent drinks of diluted fruit juice or water.

3 If your child has any fever, reduce it by giving her paracetamol or ibuprofen.

4 Pay close attention to hygiene. The infection could spread throughout the family if your child doesn't wash her hands after going to the toilet, or if you don't wash yours after changing her nappies.

Should I seek medical help?

Seek medical advice as soon as possible if your child has diarrhoea with fever and vomiting, or if she still has diarrhoea after 12 hours (six hours in babies), or if the stools are greasy, or contain mucus or blood.

What might the doctor do?

✳ A powder containing glucose and essential minerals to be added to drinks may be

prescribed. Your doctor will recommend bed-rest and a liquid diet until any fever has passed. As a rough guide, your child should drink at least 200ml (7fl oz) of liquid per kilogram (2lb) body weight in 24 hours while she has diarrhoea.

✳ For a bottlefed baby, you will probably be advised to replace milk feeds with a glucose and mineral solution, then slowly reintroduce milk. If your baby is breastfed, keep on breastfeeding.

What can I do to help?

✳ Be meticulous about hygiene.

✳ When the diarrhoea has cleared up, introduce bland foods such as yogurt and jellies.

SEE ALSO:

ENCOPRESIS (p. 104)

FEVER (p. 26)

FOOD POISONING (p. 99)

INFLUENZA (p. 87)

VOMITING (p. 100)

Constipation

Constipation is a word used to describe the consistency of stools, not the regularity or frequency of bowel movements. During babyhood, constipation is unlikely for either breastfed or bottlefed babies. When they start on solid food, however, they can suffer from it if their diet doesn't contain enough fresh fruit, vegetables, and liquids. Even if the baby's stools are hard and dry when, because of illness, she is feverish or has been vomiting, this is not true constipation. The body compensates for loss of fluid from vomiting or fever by absorbing water from the stools, and bowel activity should return to normal when the illness has passed.

Possible symptoms

* Hard pebble-like stools
* Pain in the lower abdomen
* Blood on nappy or underpants

Is it serious?

Occasional constipation is not serious and can be avoided by means of a diet rich in fibre. Chronic constipation can be serious. Blood in the stools should always be cause for concern.

How is it treated?

What should I do first?
1 If your child strains when passing stools and complains of pain, check the consistency of the stools she has passed.

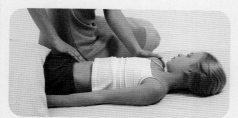

2 If your child has stomach pain and it is worse on the right side of her abdomen, check below her navel for symptoms of possible appendicitis. Consult your doctor immediately if you suspect she has appendicitis.

Should I seek medical help?
Seek medical advice immediately if your child complains of pain when moving her bowels. Consult the doctor immediately if you notice blood on your child's nappy or underpants – the passing of a large, dry stool may have injured her anal passage, a complaint that is called anal fissure.

What might the doctor do?
* Your doctor may prescribe a mild laxative that is safe to give your child for short periods.

* If an anal fissure is suspected, your doctor will examine your child's rectum, and if there is a tiny crack, he will gently lubricate the anal passage to help the skin to heal.

What can I do to help?
* Only give a laxative if the doctor advises it.

* Include as many natural, unprocessed foods as possible in his diet, with some fibre in the form of whole grains, and fresh fruit and vegetables. Don't just scatter bran over his meals; this can deplete certain minerals in the diet. A few stewed prunes or dried figs though, can produce a soft stool within 24 hours.

* Make sure your child drinks plenty of fluids.

SEE ALSO:
APPENDICITIS (p. 106), **ENCOPRESIS** (p. 104)

Encopresis

If a child frequently soils his underpants after he has been toilet trained, he is suffering from encopresis. In a child of four or five, uncontrollable bowel motions should be regarded as a symptom of a problem, rather than of slow development. The most common cause of encopresis is chronic constipation, in which hard, dry stools accumulate in the bowel, and loose, watery motions trickle out past them. You may even mistake this condition for diarrhoea. The problem often starts as the result of some emotional disturbance in the child's life, such as the arrival of a new baby, separation of parents, or moving house and losing contact with friends. Occasionally,

children persist in soiling their pants from infancy onwards. This soiling may be a reaction against over-fussy toilet training.

Is it serious?

Encopresis is not a serious problem.

Possible symptoms

* Involuntary bowel motions after the child has been toilet trained
* Chronic constipation

How is it treated?

What should I do first?
1 Try to determine whether your child is constipated. Ask him when he last went to the toilet.

2 Check whether your child is affected by any stress, such as the arrival of a new baby, moving house, or starting school.

Should I seek medical help?
Seek medical advice as soon as possible if you think your child has chronic constipation. If you can find no reason for the involuntary soiling, your doctor may be the best person to discover a possible cause of tension.

What might the doctor do?
* If your child is constipated, your doctor will prescribe a mild laxative, specially formulated for babies and children, which is safe for short-term use.

* Your doctor or health visitor will advise you on how to reduce the constipation in the future.

* If there is some emotional reason for the encopresis, your doctor will assess the situation after discussion with you and your child. If further investigation is needed, your doctor or health visitor may refer you and your child to a child psychologist.

What can I do to help?
* Make sure your child has a diet rich in dietary fibre and liquids.

* Don't punish your child or show disgust if he soils his pants; this will make the condition worse.

* Watch for signs of poor school performance. Your child may become a target of scorn because of the odour if he soils himself at school. Provide him with spare underpants.

SEE ALSO:
CONSTIPATION (p. 103)
DIARRHOEA (p. 102)

Hernia

A hernia results when a small defect in the muscular wall of the abdomen allows soft tissue to protrude through. This appears as a slight bulge in the skin, and can be seen even more clearly if your child coughs or strains. The most common type of hernia in children is umbilical hernia. This appears near the navel, and results from a weakness that occurs in the abdominal wall at birth. An inguinal hernia appears lower down in the groin and is most common in boys, the defect occurring after the testicles have descended into the scrotum. Umbilical hernias rarely need any treatment and heal themselves spontaneously. Inguinal hernias may also heal without treatment but may need to be corrected by minor surgery.

Is it serious?

A hernia is not usually serious unless the bowel is trapped.

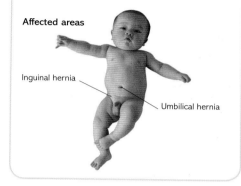

Possible symptoms

* Vomiting with sharp abdominal pain if the bowel has become trapped

* Painless bulge in the skin's surface near the navel or in the groin; the bulge increases in size when the child coughs, sneezes, or cries

Affected areas

Inguinal hernia

Umbilical hernia

How is it treated?

What should I do first?
Try to push the hernia carefully inwards. Most hernias respond to gentle pressure by sliding back inside the muscular wall.

Should I seek medical help?
Seek medical advice if you notice a bulge in your baby's abdomen before he is six months old. Consult your doctor immediately if a hernia becomes hard, and the bulge won't go back with the application of gentle pressure, and if there is accompanying vomiting and abdominal pain.

What might the doctor do?
If the hernia is hard or won't go back, your doctor will refer you to a paediatric specialist, as it will probably have to be repaired surgically.

The operation for a hernia repair is simple. If your child has an inguinal hernia, your doctor may recommend surgical repair to avoid any trapping of the bowel.

What can I do to help?
* Check an umbilical hernia regularly, at bathtimes, for example, to make sure that the hernia is not enlarging, that it is not hard, and that it goes back when gently pushed.

* Discuss future action with your doctor and decide together whether to let the hernia heal spontaneously or whether surgery is necessary.

* Take your child for regular check-ups.

SEE ALSO:

CONSTIPATION (p. 103)

DIARRHOEA (p. 102)

Appendicitis

Appendicitis occurs when the appendix becomes partly or wholly blocked, and a build-up of bacteria causes an infection. The appendix then becomes inflamed and swollen, and may need to be removed surgically. An appendectomy is a common emergency operation among children. However, appendicitis in babies under the age of 12 months is rare.

Is it serious?

If appendicitis is diagnosed early, it is not a serious condition. However, if treatment is delayed for any reason, the build-up of pus in the blocked appendix can cause it to burst. This condition may lead to peritonitis. Peritonitis is inflammation of the abdominal cavity, or peritoneum, due to bacteria in the bloodstream, and requires immediate attention.

Possible symptoms

✳ Abdominal pain, starting around the navel, then moving down to the lower right abdomen

✳ Slight temperature, rarely above 38°C (100.4°F)

✳ Loss of appetite

✳ Vomiting, diarrhoea, or constipation

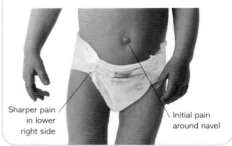

Sharper pain in lower right side

Initial pain around navel

How is it treated?

What should I do first?

1 If your child complains of an abdominal pain for more than a couple of hours, carefully lay her flat on her back. Gently press her stomach a few centimetres to the right of, and just below, the navel. If she experiences any pain on this gentle pressure, and a sharp pain when you suddenly remove your hands, these could both be signs of appendicitis. Consult your doctor immediately.

2 If your child is constipated and you suspect appendicitis, don't give her laxatives; they can cause an inflamed appendix to burst.

3 Don't give your child anything to eat or drink in case an appendectomy is necessary.

Should I seek medical help?

Seek medical advice immediately, as delay could allow the appendix to burst and cause peritonitis.

What might the doctor do?

Your doctor will examine your child's abdomen and ask you to describe symptoms. Your child may need to be admitted to hospital to confirm the diagnosis, and for surgical removal of the appendix, if necessary.

What can I do to help?

✳ Arrange to stay with your child at the hospital overnight.

✳ Encourage your child to rest and eat normally when she returns home from hospital, usually the day after the operation. Your child should recover fully after two to three weeks.

SEE ALSO:
CONSTIPATION (p. 103)

Chapter 7

Muscles, bones, and joints

In growing children, the muscles, bones, and joints are still developing and are therefore particularly vulnerable to injury. This chapter concentrates on recognizing symptoms and dealing with them.

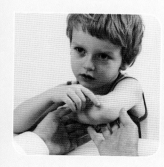
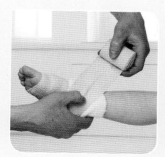
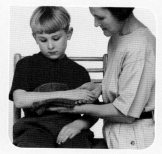

Diagnosis guide

Most muscle, bone, and joint problems in young children are easily spotted. Some, however, are difficult to diagnose accurately. If in doubt, always consult your doctor, or take your child to the nearest hospital emergency department. To use this section, look for the symptom most similar to the one your child is suffering from, then turn to the relevant entry. See also p. 13 for a list of symptoms requiring emergency treatment.

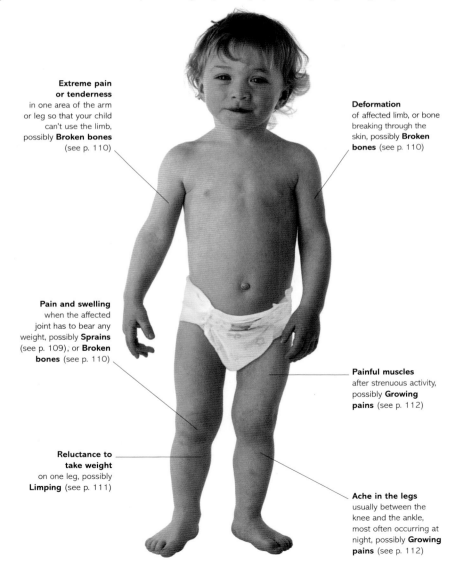

Extreme pain or tenderness
in one area of the arm or leg so that your child can't use the limb, possibly **Broken bones** (see p. 110)

Deformation
of affected limb, or bone breaking through the skin, possibly **Broken bones** (see p. 110)

Pain and swelling
when the affected joint has to bear any weight, possibly **Sprains** (see p. 109), or **Broken bones** (see p. 110)

Painful muscles
after strenuous activity, possibly **Growing pains** (see p. 112)

Reluctance to take weight
on one leg, possibly **Limping** (see p. 111)

Ache in the legs
usually between the knee and the ankle, most often occurring at night, possibly **Growing pains** (see p. 112)

Sprains

A sprain is the tearing of the tough, strap-like structures (ligaments) that support a joint and limit its movement. The sprain usually occurs because of overstretching or a sudden twisting action that wrenches the joint beyond its normal range of movement. The tearing causes bleeding into the joint, which results in swelling, pain, and a bad bruise.

The most common sites of a sprain are the ankle, knee, and wrist. Because the ligaments are near the skin's surface in these joints, swelling shows rapidly, and your child finds it difficult to take any weight on the sprained joint.

It is rare for young children to suffer a sprain because their joints are highly supple. Sprains are, however, quite common in the six to 12-year-old age group.

Are they serious?
A sprain can be painful, but it is not serious. Because it can be difficult to determine without an X-ray whether the injury is a sprain, a broken bone, or a dislocated joint, it is always sensible to seek medical help for an accurate diagnosis.

Possible symptoms

* Swelling and tenderness
* Pain when the affected joint has to bear any weight
* Bruising

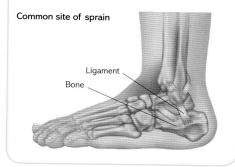

Common site of sprain

Ligament
Bone

How are they treated?

What should I do first?
1 If the affected joint or limb is not misshapen, lay your child down, and raise the injured part.

2 Apply a cold compress to reduce the swelling.

3 Support the joint with a firm crepe bandage applied over a thick wad of cotton wool. Check the bandage regularly to make sure that subsequent swelling has not made it too tight.

4 Encourage your child to rest the joint for at least 24 hours.

Should I seek medical help?
Take your child to the nearest hospital emergency department if there is intense pain and the affected joint or limb is misshapen, or if after 48 hours the swelling has not subsided or if your child still complains of severe pain and cannot bear any weight on the injured part.

What might the doctor do?
The emergency department staff will assess the injury, X-ray if necessary, and advise on further care.

SEE ALSO:
BROKEN BONES (p. 110)

Broken bones

Children's bones do not break as easily as the harder bones of an adult. The most common fracture in children is the greenstick fracture, where the bone bends rather than breaks, and where there is minimal damage to the surrounding tissues. In a closed fracture, the bone breaks at one place and does not break the skin. In an open fracture, the bone ends stick through the skin, and may damage blood vessels and muscles.

Possible symptoms

✳ Swelling and bruising around the site of the injury

✳ Possible deformity of the affected area

✳ Inability to move the affected area normally

✳ Pain

Are they serious?

A broken bone should always be treated promptly by a doctor for various reasons. It has to be set correctly, and any damage to surrounding organs or tissues has to be repaired. There is also a risk of infection if the break is an open fracture, and the bone is exposed to the air.

How are they treated?

What should I do first?

1 Dial 999/112 for emergency help if the injury involves your child's leg or elbow. Otherwise, take your child to hospital.

2 If the limb appears bent or curved, don't try to straighten it. Don't move your child unless you have to. If a bone has broken through the skin, or if there is a wound leading down to the fracture, drape a sterile dressing over it. Don't attempt any cleaning, and don't touch the wound.

3 If no bone is sticking through the skin, but he cannot move the affected area without causing pain, immobilize above and below the break: put an arm in a sling; for a leg, tie the knees and the ankles together. Take him to the nearest hospital, but call an ambulance if the legs or elbows are affected because you will need a stretcher.

4 Don't give your child anything to eat and drink in case he needs surgery.

5 Keep him warm and calm while you get medical help. Try to raise the affected part after immobilizing it.

Should I seek medical advice?

Dial 999/112 for emergency help if the bone is bent or curved, if it is sticking through the skin, or if a leg or elbow is broken. If you suspect your child has another broken bone, take him to the nearest emergency department.

What might the doctor do?

✳ The doctor will X-ray your child to determine the extent of the damage. With a straightforward break, the bone will be immobilized by setting it in a plaster of Paris cast.

✳ If the break is an open fracture, the bones will be manipulated into position under a general anaesthetic before being immobilized in plaster.

✳ If there is an open wound with the broken bone, antibiotics will be given.

✳ If the child has had a bad break in his leg, he may have to remain in hospital in traction.

What can I do to help?

Make sure the plaster cast is kept dry. Broken bones in children heal within six to 10 weeks.

Limping

Your child is limping if he is not taking the full weight of his body on one leg then the other as he walks. The cause may be obvious, such as a cut, a blister, or a splinter on the sole of the foot, an ingrowing toenail, a pebble in a shoe, or tight shoes.

Is it serious?

A persistent limp that seems to have no apparent reason should always be treated promptly in a child since it may be a symptom of a more serious problem. You should always consult your doctor if your child limps. An unexplained limp can be a symptom of a form of blood cancer, leukaemia. If the limp is accompanied by any swelling or tenderness of the joints, this could be caused by rheumatic fever, arthritis, or osteomyelitis. All of these diseases could have long-term complications, so it is recommended to get your child's limp treated as soon as possible.

How is it treated?

What should I do first?
1 Look for obvious injuries and examine any areas that your child claims are painful.

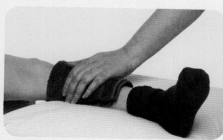

2 Check if the joints are swollen or inflamed.

3 If you suspect your child may have a broken bone in his foot or toe, don't hesitate to get medical attention. If a bone in his leg is affected, dial 999/112 for emergency help. The injury may not always be obvious.

Should I seek medical help?
Seek medical advice and a thorough examination of the limp if you can't find a reason for it. If you suspect a broken bone, either dial 999/112 for emergency help or take your child to the nearest hospital emergency department. Consult your doctor if any of your child's joints are swollen or tender.

What might the doctor do?
Your doctor will examine your child's leg thoroughly, and may refer him to a paediatric orthopaedic surgeon to find the cause of the problem.

What can I do to help?
Never give up if your child has an unexplained limp. Be persistent until the cause is identified and treated appropriately.

SEE ALSO:

BLISTERS (p. 41)

BROKEN BONES (p. 110)

CUTS AND GRAZES (p. 36)

INGROWING TOENAILS (p. 59)

SPLINTERS (p. 39)

Growing pains

A growing pain is a dull, vague ache in a limb; it doesn't last for long, and the child can usually be distracted from it. One in six children of school age suffers from some kind of growing pain. Such pains can occur when your child is going through a growth spurt, during which the muscles and bones grow at slightly different rates, leading to an aching soreness that is worse in the evening. Growing pains can also occur after a strenuous activity. It is important to distinguish a growing pain from a joint pain. A growing pain is felt between the joints of a limb, while a joint pain is specific to the joint area. In a child, a joint pain can be a symptom of rheumatic fever or arthritis.

Possible symptoms

✳ Aches and pains in the arms or legs, most often in the legs

✳ Disturbed sleep if the pain is severe

✳ Painful muscles after strenuous activity

accompanied by a fever. This could be septic arthritis. You should consult your doctor as soon as possible if your child has these symptoms.

Are they serious?

A growing pain is not serious, but any pain in the joint could be, particularly if it is

How are they treated?

What should I do first?

1 Check your child's joints for swelling and tenderness by pressing on and around them. If there is neither, check the muscles in the same way.

2 Check to see if your child limps when she walks.

3 Ask your child when the pain started and for how long it lasts.

Should I seek medical help?

Seek medical advice as soon as possible if the pain is sited around a joint and is accompanied by a fever, or if it lasts for longer than 24 hours.

What might the doctor do?

After excluding any other possible causes of the pain, your doctor will reassure you

and your child that there is no cause for you to be concerned.

What can I do to help?

✳ Show sympathetic interest in the pain – this may be sufficient to relax your child.

✳ Give your child a warm bath before she goes to bed. You can also give her a hot-water bottle to take to bed. Both of these can be very soothing if your child is having difficulty sleeping.

✳ Gently massage the affected muscles to relax any tension.

SEE ALSO:

FEVER (p. 26)

LIMPING (p. 111)

Chapter 8

Head
and brain

The nervous system is made up of the
brain and the spinal cord, and millions of
interconnecting nerve cells. Background
information and advice on common diseases
of the nervous system is given here.

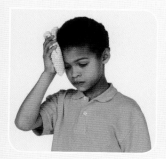

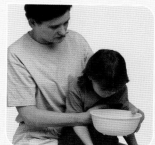

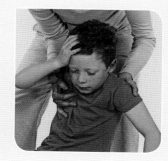

Diagnosis guide

Children find it difficult to describe pain; they may simply appear "ill". A hand held to the head may signify a headache, so never hesitate to contact your doctor for clarification. Check your baby's temperature – any headache accompanied by fever is serious. To use this section, look for the signs most similar to the ones that your child has, then turn to the relevant entry. See also p. 13 for a list of symptoms requiring emergency treatment.

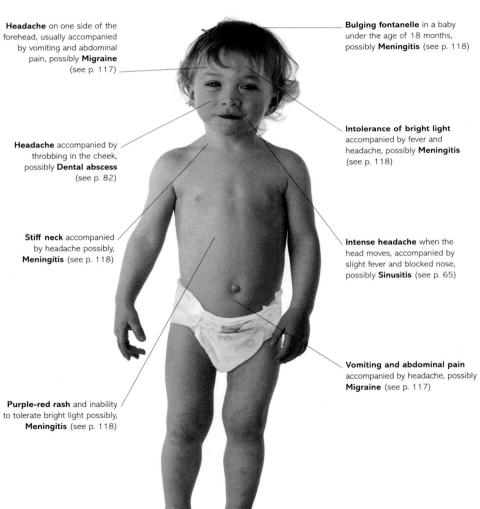

Headache on one side of the forehead, usually accompanied by vomiting and abdominal pain, possibly **Migraine** (see p. 117)

Headache accompanied by throbbing in the cheek, possibly **Dental abscess** (see p. 82)

Stiff neck accompanied by headache possibly, **Meningitis** (see p. 118)

Purple-red rash and inability to tolerate bright light possibly, **Meningitis** (see p. 118)

Bulging fontanelle in a baby under the age of 18 months, possibly **Meningitis** (see p. 118)

Intolerance of bright light accompanied by fever and headache, possibly **Meningitis** (see p. 118)

Intense headache when the head moves, accompanied by slight fever and blocked nose, possibly **Sinusitis** (see p. 65)

Vomiting and abdominal pain accompanied by headache, possibly **Migraine** (see p. 117)

Dizziness

Dizziness describes a feeling of unsteadiness and spinning about. When a child is out of breath, she may feel a bit dizzy because there is a less than normal supply of oxygen to her brain. Your child may also feel dizzy if she is suffering from anaemia (a shortage of iron in the blood). A bang on the head that results in loss of consciousness, or a seizure, may be preceded by dizziness. However, under normal circumstances, dizziness should usually clear up within two or three minutes.

Is it serious?

Momentary dizziness is not serious, but if dizzy spells last longer than 12 hours, they may be caused by anaemia.

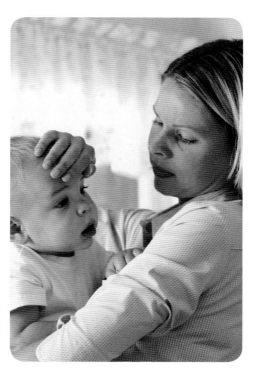

Soothing your baby Dizzy spells can be very distressing for your baby. Try to keep her quiet and calm by holding her close to you and soothing her.

How is it treated?

What should I do first?
1 Lay your child down and prop her legs up on some cushions. This increases the flow of blood, and therefore oxygen, to her brain. Loosen any tight clothing and tell her to take a few deep breaths.

2 Keep her quiet and calm if that is what she wants.

3 Note how long she says the dizzy feeling lasts.

Should I seek medical help?
Seek medical advice if your child experiences dizzy spells over a 12-hour period but has no other symptoms. Check with your doctor as soon as possible if your child is continually complaining of dizziness after strenuous activity; this may be a sign of anaemia.

What might the doctor do?
After examining your child, your doctor will determine the cause of the dizziness. If the dizziness is a symptom of a more serious disorder, such as anaemia, your doctor will treat this accordingly.

Headache

About one in five children suffers from recurrent headaches, although a serious physical cause is hardly ever found. Most commonly, children complain of pain in their heads after sitting in a hot, stuffy room, if they are worried or anxious about something, if they have a fever, or they have sinusitis or toothache, for example. Some children complain frequently of headache and stomach ache. Such pain is known as abdominal migraine. If your child has had a recent injury to his head, and continues to have headaches, you should seek immediate medical attention.

Is it serious?

Headaches are rarely serious, but if a single headache is accompanied by a fever, neck stiffness, confusion, or an intolerance of bright light, this may be a symptom of a more serious illness, such as meningitis, and you should seek medical advice immediately.

How is it treated?

What should I do first?

1 Ask your child if he has pain anywhere else. Run your hands over the area around his cheeks, jaw, and ears to see if sinusitis, a dental abscess, toothache, or earache is the problem.

2 Check his temperature to see if he has a fever. Headache and fever could be among the first symptoms of an infectious illness, such as influenza.

3 Check to see if your child has any injury to his head.

4 If the headaches are frequent, find out if your child is worried about anything, such as his school work.

5 If he complains of nausea or vomits, this could be a migraine headache.

6 If he has no other symptoms to concern you, give him a dose of paracetamol or ibuprofen to relieve the pain, and put him to bed in a darkened room for half an hour.

Should I seek medical help?

Seek medical advice immediately if the headache is accompanied by a temperature of 38°C (100.4°F) with vomiting, neck stiffness, and intolerance of bright light, if your child has had a recent head injury, or if headaches are persistent.

What might the doctor do?

✳ Your doctor will examine your child. This may include taking your child's blood pressure, and looking at the retina in the eye. Further tests will be carried out only if your doctor finds something wrong apart from the headaches.

✳ If the headache is a symptom of a more serious condition, your doctor will treat the condition accordingly.

What can I do to help?

If your child complains of a headache at the end of a school day, give him a drink and a nutritious snack, and encourage him to go out and play in the fresh air.

SEE ALSO:

EARACHE (p. 70), **FEVER** (p. 26), **DENTAL ABSCESS** (p. 82), **INFLUENZA** (p. 87), **MEASLES** (p. 28), **MENINGITIS** (p. 118), **MIGRAINE** (p. 117), **SINUSITIS** (p. 65), **TOOTHACHE** (p. 80)

Migraine

Migraine is a severe, recurrent headache (felt on one or both sides of the head) that is often accompanied by vomiting and, in children, by abdominal pain. For this reason, childhood migraine can sometimes be referred to as abdominal migraine. Migraine tends to run in families, and usually starts in late childhood or in early adolescence. Headaches in children who are younger than this are not usually migraine headaches. It is not yet known what sets off a typical migraine attack, but tension and certain foods, such as chocolate, citrus fruit, and cheese, are all possible culprits. Quite often a migraine headache is preceded by an "aura", a series of strange sensations, such as flashing lights, peculiar smells, and numbness on the affected side of the head. Most children can pinpoint these sensations quite clearly.

Possible symptoms

* Severe headache on one or both sides
* Vomiting
* Nausea
* Abdominal pain
* Paleness
* Withdrawn, quiet behaviour
* Aura, involving strange visual and physical sensations, preceding the attack

Is it serious?

Migraine is not serious, but it is debilitating. Do seek medical advice if your child suffers recurrent migraine attacks.

How is it treated?

What should I do first?

1 Put your child to bed in a cool, darkened room if he complains of headache and nausea. If the headache persists, it is best to give him a dose of liquid paracetamol or ibuprofen.

2 Put a bucket next to your child's bed so that he can vomit without worrying about getting to the toilet in time.

3 If your child is complaining of abdominal pain, check him for signs of appendicitis.

Should I seek medical help?

Seek medical advice immediately if your child is suffering from severe abdominal pains, to exclude the possibility of appendicitis. Check with your doctor as soon as possible if your child suffers from recurrent migraine headaches.

What might the doctor do?

Your doctor will ask your child to describe the headache. Your doctor may prescribe painkilling drugs for an acute attack. If your child's headaches are frequent, he may be given drugs to take immediately after an attack begins or, in severe cases, to be taken regularly to prevent attacks.

What can I do to help?

If the headaches are frequent, keep a diary of your child's diet to try to pinpoint a possible trigger food. Avoid any suspect foods for a couple of weeks to see if there is any reduction in the headaches.

SEE ALSO:

APPENDICITIS (p. 106)

HEADACHE (p. 116)

VOMITING (p. 100)

Meningitis

Meningitis is an inflammation of the membranes (meninges) that cover the brain and spinal cord, and most frequently results from an infection, either viral or bacterial. Any meningitis is serious, but can be treated successfully with antibiotics if it is diagnosed early enough. The symptoms of meningitis are fever, stiff neck, lethargy, headache, drowsiness, intolerance of bright light, cold hands and feet, joint and limb pain, and mottled or pale skin; in rare cases, there may also be a purple-red rash. Meningitis can be difficult to diagnose in babies and very young children, because they are unable to communicate what they are feeling. However, under 18 months old, one noticeable symptom is that the fontanelle will bulge slightly. The fontanelle is the soft part of the skull. If your child is suffering from bacterial meningitis, she will be given high doses of antibiotics intravenously. Viral meningitis clears up on its own, but your child may be given painkilling drugs to relieve the symptoms.

Is it serious?

Meningitis is very serious and, if left untreated, it can prove fatal.

Possible symptoms

* ✳ Fever, as high as 39°C (102.2°F)
* ✳ Stiff neck
* ✳ Lethargy, headache, drowsiness, and confusion
* ✳ Inability to tolerate bright light
* ✳ Bulging fontanelle in babies
* ✳ Vomiting
* ✳ Purple-red rash anywhere on the body
* ✳ Cold hands and feet
* ✳ Joint and limb pain
* ✳ Mottled or pale skin

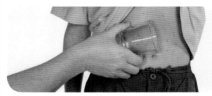

Checking rash
Check for a rash, which doesn't fade when pressed with a glass. If present, dial 999/112 for emergency help and insist on being seen at once.

How is it treated?

What should I do first?

1 If you suspect meningitis, bend your child's head forward so that her chin touches her chest to see if there is any stiffness in her neck.

2 If your child is under two years old, check to see if she screws her eyes up in bright light. Feel the fontanelle to see if it bulges outwards.

3 If your child has a purple-red rash anywhere on her body, press a glass against it. If the rash does not fade, call for emergency help at once.

Should I seek medical help?
Seek medical advice immediately if you suspect meningitis or dial 999/112 for emergency help.

What might the doctor do?
If meningitis is suspected, your child will go to hospital for a lumbar puncture. This involves removing a sample of spinal fluid for examination.

SEE ALSO:
FEVER (p. 26)
HEADACHE (p. 116)

Chapter 9

Urinary and genital infections

Urinary and genital infections are common in childhood. They can be distressing but most clear up quickly. This chapter covers two of the most common problems, thrush and balanitis.

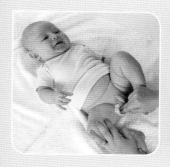
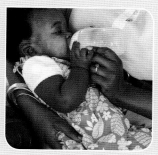
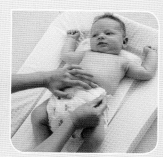

Diagnosis guide

Minor infections of the genitals are quite common in young children and, although they can be distressing, they are not usually serious. To use this section, look for the symptom most similar to the one your child is suffering from, then turn to the relevant entry. See also p. 13 for a list of symptoms requiring emergency treatment.

Boys' genitals

By the time your son is about three or four, the foreskin will be loose and will retract easily. Before that age, you should never try to pull it back for cleaning; just wash the penis carefully. Try to encourage your son to wash the genital area gently from front to back.

Girls' genitals

Careful hygiene can prevent many genital problems. Teach your little girl to wipe her bottom from front to back so that bacteria from the rectum do not infect the vagina. Scented soap or bubble bath can cause irritation of the genital area, so use mild, unscented products.

Pain or itching in the genital area, possibly **Balanitis** (see p. 122)

Foreskin that cannot be drawn back, possibly **Balanitis** (see p. 122)

Red, swollen tip of the penis, possibly **Balanitis** (see p. 122)

Red, inflamed buttocks and genital region, possibly **Nappy rash** (see p. 49) or **Balanitis** (see p. 122)

Pimply red rash on the area normally covered by your baby's nappy, possibly **Thrush** (see p. 121) or **Nappy rash** (see p. 49)

Thrush

Thrush is a common infection caused by the fungus *Candida albicans*. Under normal circumstances, this fungus is kept under control by other bacteria that also live in the intestines. However, if the balance is disturbed for any reason – for example, when your child is on a course of antibiotics, or his natural resistance is low because of disease – the fungus can grow unchecked, causing infection in any part of the gastrointestinal tract.

Thrush most often affects the mouth. It can also affect the anus. In babies, anal thrush is sometimes confused with nappy rash. Unlike nappy rash, however, it does not respond to the usual home treatments.

Possible symptoms

* For oral thrush, creamy yellow or white frothy patches inside the cheeks, on the tongue, and the roof of the mouth, which become raw or bleed when wiped off
* A pimply, red rash around the anus

Is it serious?

Thrush is rarely serious, but if it does not respond to home treatment, get help. It's important to treat anal thrush both orally and topically or it usually recurs.

How is it treated?

What should I do first?

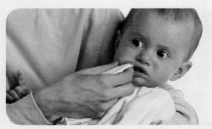

1 If your child refuses to eat, check his mouth for any white patches. Try to wipe them off with a clean handkerchief. If they don't come off or if they leave raw patches underneath, he probably has oral thrush.

2 Avoid giving your child spicy foods, and cool all cooked food to lukewarm temperature. Natural yogurt is the best food to give until you have consulted your doctor.

3 Change your baby's nappies frequently. The fungus may be in his stools, and this could give rise to thrush around the anus.

Should I seek medical help?
Seek medical advice if you suspect your child has thrush.

What might the doctor do?
* Your doctor will prescribe a liquid antifungal medication to be dropped on to the affected area in your child's mouth if he has oral thrush.

* Your doctor will prescribe an antifungal cream if there is a rash around the anus.

What can I do to help?
* Feed your child with mild, liquidized foods if he has oral thrush.

* Keep your child's hands clean so that the infection does not spread from the anus to the mouth, or vice versa.

* Leave your baby's bottom exposed to the air as much as possible if he is still in nappies.

SEE ALSO:
NAPPY RASH (p. 49)

Balanitis

Balanitis is the inflammation of the tip (glans) of the penis. It may be caused by nappy rash, by an allergic reaction to the soap powder in which your child's clothes are washed, or by a tight foreskin in boys aged three to five years (phimosis) – up until then, the foreskin is normally tight.

Is it serious?

The condition is not serious, although it is important for your son's comfort that you treat the condition promptly. If it is recurrent, he may need to be circumcised.

Possible symptoms

- ✳ Red, swollen, moist tip of the penis
- ✳ Discharge of pus from the tip of the penis
- ✳ A foreskin that cannot be drawn back
- ✳ If your child is still in nappies, a general inflammation around the buttocks and in the genital region

How is it treated?

What should I do first?

1 As soon as you notice any redness around the tip of the penis, gently try to draw back the foreskin. Don't force it, and leave it if your son is under five. If the foreskin won't retract, leave it alone and consult your doctor.

2 If the foreskin will retract, wash and dry the penis and apply an antiseptic ointment.

3 If the condition is part of nappy rash, change your child's nappies frequently, wash and dry the area thoroughly at every nappy change, and apply a barrier cream liberally over the area covered by the nappy, including the penis.

Should I seek medical help?

Seek medical advice if your child complains of pain, if you cannot retract the foreskin, or if home treatment fails to relieve the swelling within 48 hours.

What might the doctor do?

✳ Your child may be prescribed an antibiotic cream to relieve the inflammation of the penis.

✳ If the foreskin is tight, your doctor will regularly check on it; if the foreskin has failed

to stretch by the time your son is six years old, the condition may need to be corrected surgically by circumcision. Your doctor will refer you to a paediatrician who will assess your child to see if he really needs to be circumcised.

What can I do to help?

✳ Always change your child's nappies frequently to prevent the recurrence of nappy rash.

✳ Teach your child good personal hygiene from an early age. Up until the age of five regular bathing will keep the penis adequately cleaned. After this age, encourage your child to draw back the foreskin and wash the area every day.

✳ If an allergic reaction has caused balanitis, try changing your washing powder, and make sure that your child's clothing is thoroughly rinsed.

SEE ALSO:

NAPPY RASH (p. 49)

Useful addresses

Action for Sick Children
32b Buxton Road
High Lane
Stockport SK6 8BH
Tel: 01663 763 004
www.actionforsickchildren.org
*Pressure group that seeks to
raise awareness about the welfare
of sick children*

British Dyslexia Association
Unit 8 Bracknell Beeches
Old Bracknell Lane
Bracknell RG12 7BW
Tel: 0845 251 9002
www.bdadyslexia.org.uk
Email: helpline@bdadyslexia.org.uk

British Red Cross
UK Office
44 Moorfields
London EC2Y 9AL
Tel: 0844 871 1111
www.redcross.org.uk

British Stammering Association
15 Old Ford Road
London E2 9PJ
Tel: 020 8983 1003
www.stammering.org
Email: mail@stammering.org

Contact-a-Family
209-211 City Road
London EC1V 1JN
Tel: 0808 808 3555
www.cafamily.org.uk
Email: helpline@cafamily.org.uk
*Puts parents of children with special
needs in touch with others in their
area for support*

MENCAP (The Royal Society
for Mentally Handicapped
Children and Adults)
123 Golden Lane
London EC1Y 0RT
Tel: 020 7454 0454
www.mencap.org.uk
Email: information@mencap.org.uk
For people with learning disabilities

The National Association
for Gifted Children (NAGC)
Suite 14 Challenge House
Sherwood Drive
Bletchley
Milton Keynes MK3 6DP
Tel: 0845 450 0295
www.nagcbritain.org.uk
Email: amazingchildren@nagcbritain.
org.uk

The National Deaf
Children's Society
15 Dufferin Street
London EC1Y 8UR
Tel: 0808 800 8880
www.ndcs.org.uk
Email: ndcs@ndcs.org.uk

The National Eczema Society
Hill House
Highgate Hill
London N19 5NA
Helpline: 0800 0891122
www.eczema.org
Email: helpline@eczema.org

Royal National Institute
for the Blind (RNIB)
105 Judd Street
London WC1H 9NE
Tel: 020 7388 1266
www.rnib.org.uk
Email: helpline@rnib.org.uk

St Andrew's Ambulance
Association
St Andrew's House
48 Milton Street
Glasgow G4 0HR
Tel: 0141 332 4031
www.firstaid.org.uk

St John Ambulance
27 St. John's Lane
London EC1M 4BU
Tel: 0870 010 4950
www.sja.org.uk

Child Accident Prevention Trust
4th Floor, Cloister Court
22-26 Farringdon Lane
London EC1R 3AJ
Tel: 020 7608 3828
www.capt.org.uk
Email: safe@capt.org.uk

Royal Society for the Prevention
of Accidents (RoSPA)
Edgbaston Park
353 Bristol Road
Birmingham B5 7ST
Tel: 0121 248 2000
www.rospa.com
Email: help@rospa.com

Foundation for the Study
of Infant Deaths
Artillery House
11-19 Artillery Row
London SW1P 1RT
Tel: 020 7233 2090
www.sids.org.uk/fsid
Available 24 hours

Glossary

Acute
A term applied to short attacks of a disease or pain.

Allergen
Any substance that provokes an allergic reaction in certain individuals.

Anaesthetic
A drug used to bring about temporary loss of sensation and hence remove pain. General anaesthetics induce unconsciousness, and are given in the form of an injection or through inhalation, usually for more serious surgical procedures. Local anaesthetics are usually given as injections and remove sensation from only a limited area. They are used primarily for minor but painful operations.

Analgesic
A pain-relieving drug. The one most frequently given to children is paracetamol, which is available in liquid and tablet forms. The liquid comes in two strengths: infant, from three months to six years, and junior, from six to 12 years.

Antibiotic
A drug used to fight bacterial infection. A prescribed course should always be completed, even if the illness is cured.

Antifungal
A drug used to treat fungal infections, such as thrush or athlete's foot.

Antihistamine
A drug used to counter the effects of histamines, chemicals produced by the body as a result of an allergic, inflammatory reaction. Antihistamine drugs are used to treat illnesses, such as hives.

Autoimmune
A defect in the body's defence system against disease, which causes the body to manufacture antibodies that attack and harm its own healthy tissue.

Bacteria
A group of organisms, some of which are harmless and some only harmful when they multiply too quickly. Harmful bacteria can cause illnesses, such as food poisoning and tonsillitis.

Bronchodilator
A drug that widens bronchial passages, and is used in the treatment of asthma. It is taken either by nasal inhalation or orally through a spray.

Chronic
A term describing a condition that has lasted, or is expected to last, for some time, while not necessarily being life-threatening.

CPR
Cardiopulmonary resuscitation – a combination of rescue breaths and chest compressions.

Excretion
The removal of the body's internal waste matter by natural processes, such as urination and sweating.

Follicle
Most commonly, a tiny cavity on the body's surface.

Hormone
A chemical released by the endocrine glands into the bloodstream. It regulates the activities of certain body organs and tissues.

Immunization
The process by which the body is prepared, by vaccination, to repel any infection or disease.

Incubation period
The interval (measured in days) between the time a disease is caught – when the germs enter the body – and when symptoms appear.

Infection
A type of illness caused by microbes invading the body and multiplying within it. The microbes may clog up blood vessels and ducts, and can also produce harmful waste products.

Laxative
A type of drug used to ease and increase the frequency of bowel movements. They should be given to a child only on doctor's orders.

Membrane
A thin lining or tissue covering the various organs and cavities of the body.

Meninges
The three layers of membrane protecting the brain and spinal cord. Meningitis is an inflammation of the meninges.

Microbes
Minute bacteria, viruses, or fungi invisible to the naked eye.

Mucus membrane
A membrane lining a part of the body, such as the mouth or vagina, which secretes watery or slimy material.

Otoscope
An instrument used to examine the middle and inner ear, which allows

the doctor to view through the semi-transparent eardrum, to diagnose the disease.

Penicillin

The first antibiotic to be discovered, penicillin is used in the treatment of many infections, including middle ear infection and tonsillitis. It may provoke an allergic reaction. If your child is allergic, make sure this is entered on his medical records and that he wears a medic-alert bracelet so that he isn't given the drug.

Possetting

In babies, the harmless habit of regurgitating milk soon after, or during, a feed.

Pus

A yellow-green substance made up of decomposed tissue, bacteria, and dead white blood cells – it is a sign of the body's fight against infection.

Shock

A reduction of blood flow throughout the body, which, if untreated, may lead to collapse, coma, and death.

Spasm

An involuntary and uncontrollable contraction of one or more muscles.

Stools

The waste matter left over from food, expelled from the rectum.

Toxin

A poisonous substance produced by bacteria, other microbes, and some plants and animals.

Traction

A method of treating broken bones, crushed vertebrae, and prolapsed discs. The damaged and compressed parts of the body are held apart by a complex system of pulleys and weights in the correct position until healed.

Ulcer

An open sore affecting either an internal or an external body surface.

Vaccine

A solution made up of an altered, weakened, or killed strain of a disease. Usually injected, it is designed to stimulate the body's resistance to the disease that has been introduced.

Vasodilator

Any substance, whether a chemical produced by the body, or a drug, which causes blood vessels to widen.

Virus

The smallest type of microbe, which invades the body's cells and multiplies inside them, giving rise to contagious viral infections such as influenza.

Index

Acknowledgments

Medical consultant: Dr Vivien Armstrong
Proofreader: Angela Baynham

The publisher would like to thank the following
for their kind permission to reproduce their
photographs:

(Key: b-bottom; l-left; r-right)

Corbis: Lester V. Bergman 75; Edith Held
107bl; Getty Images: altrendo images 38;
Comstock Images 83bl, 86; DAJ 105; Digital

Vision 23br; Fuse 61bl; Mother & Baby
Picture Library: Ian Hooton 17; Science Photo
Library: 29; Dr P. Marazzi 53

All other images © Dorling Kindersley
For further information see:
www.dkimages.com